'While I'm here, doctor'

'While I'm here, doctor'

A study of change in the doctor–patient relationship

EDITED BY

Andrew Elder and Oliver Samuel

Foreword by Enid Balint

TAVISTOCK PUBLICATIONS

LONDON and NEW YORK

First published in 1987 by
Tavistock Publications Ltd
11 New Fetter Lane, London EC4P 4EE

Published in the USA by
Tavistock Publications
in association with Methuen, Inc.
29 West 35th Street, New York NY 10001

Printed in Great Britain by
J. W. Arrowsmith Ltd, Bristol

British Library Cataloguing in Publication Data
While I'm here, doctor: a study of change
in the doctor–patient relationship.
1. Physician and patient   2. Communication
in medicine
I. Elder, Andrew II. Samuel, Oliver
610.69'6   R727.3
ISBN 0–422–61790–3

Library of Congress Cataloging in Publication Data
"While I'm here, doctor".
Includes bibliographies and index.
1. Physician and patient—Case studies.   2. Physicians
—Psychology—Case studies.   I. Elder, Andrew, 1945–   .
II. Samuel, Oliver, 1930–   . [DNLM: 1. Physician–
Patient Relations.   2. Physicians—psychology.
W 62 W572]
R727.3.W47   1987   610.69'6   87–10200
ISBN 0–422–61790–3 (soft)

Contents

The contributors

Enid Balint is a psychoanalyst who, with her husband Michael Balint, developed training-cum-research groups for general practitioners in the early 1950s. An author and teacher of international reputation, she is an Honorary Fellow of the Royal College of General Practitioners.

Marie Campkin is in general practice in North London and is Course Organizer of the Whittington Hospital GP Vocational Training Scheme.

Andrew Elder is in group practice at the Lisson Grove Health Centre, Marylebone. He has practised there for fifteen years and is Course Organizer of the St Mary's and St Charles' GP Vocational Training Scheme. He has written on bereavement and psychotherapy in general practice.

Cyril Gill was one of the authors of *Six Minutes for the Patient* and has been involved with the development of undergraduate teaching in general practice at the Royal Free Medical School. He was a founding member and supervisor for many years at the Camden Bereavement Service. He was Secretary and then President of the Balint Society.

Erica Jones has been a general practitioner in the East End of London for many years. She is a member of the Institute of Psychosexual Medicine and is a general practice trainer.

Paul Julian is in a five-man partnership in Hackney. He is part-time Senior Lecturer in the Department of General Practice of the combined medical schools of Barts and the London Hospital.

Jack Norell was Dean of Studies of the Royal College of General Practitioners and has practised in Islington for over twenty-five years. He was co-editor of *Six Minutes for the Patient* and is the immediate past President of the Balint Society. He has written widely on medical subjects.

John Salinsky is a general practitioner in Wembley. He is treasurer of the International Balint Federation and Course Organizer of the Northwick Park GP Vocational Training Scheme.

Oliver Samuel was the first course organizer of the Northwick Park GP Vocational Training Scheme and helped to initiate the adaptation of Balint Group Training for GP Trainees. He is a general practice trainer and has worked in his practice in Harrow for almost thirty years. He has written on subjects related to medical education, notably the assessment of GP trainees.

Acknowledgements

We are greatly indebted to our patients who after all remain the principal source of education for all doctors.

The study of a particular doctor's efforts with an individual patient brings the work of a Balint group alive. Similarly in a book, it is the written description of these cases that becomes the heart of the text. We have taken care to disguise any characteristics that might easily lead to any of our patients being identified, while at the same time hoping to have preserved enough of the essence of each interaction to give an accurate account of the original. For the most part this has been done by using a slightly edited version of the doctor's own description of the case to the group. We hope very much that we have achieved this and that no embarrassment or distress is caused to any of our patients through any inadvertent recognition.

We are also grateful to the Council and members of the Balint Society who gave us continued support throughout this project, including their financial assistance with the cost of transcribing our meetings and preparing the final typescript.

Foreword

I am very glad I have been asked to write a Foreword for this book. In the Epilogue to *Six Minutes for the Patient* (1973), I said that I hoped that in our next book, we would have had the chance to clarify which kind of patient would benefit from the kind of treatment we described in that book: namely, short, brief encounters with patients over a period, during ordinary surgery hours, rather than long interviews which we had studied earlier.

This book approaches the same question by showing the variety of ways different doctors work with their more 'difficult' patients during their ordinary surgery hours. 'Long interviews' are seldom used. The book is useful and enlightening because it shows the number of ways that different doctors approach the same problems – problems which at one time we would have thought would only have been helped if the patient had been referred to a psychiatrist, psychotherapist, or by long interviews with the doctor himself at the end of the day. Each doctor in the book has his or her own style and technique, yet all have been able to work together over a number of years without trying to work out a rigid 'This is right, this is wrong' structure.

The observations made in this book take us a long way further in our ability to assess the usefulness of our work and what happens if observations are made which are usually not noticed or are bypassed. This time it is again clear that general practitioners are not being asked by psychoanalysts to become minor psychotherapists or part-time psychoanalysts, but are encouraged to use themselves and to watch themselves, to assess the way the patients are helped by them and what they need from their doctors. The role of the psychoanalyst is less obtrusive on this occasion.

Unfortunately, I was only able to participate in the first two years of the work of the group that has written this book, but their individual style of writing and thinking is well known to me, as is their openness of mind and their willingness to reconsider their own, as well as their patients' problems.

I want to assure the reader that our work of observation and discovery is not at an end. The many questions which will be in the mind of the reader when he has read this book are probably also in our minds, and we will continue to describe our voyage of discovery. I am delighted that the work which Michael Balint started still continues with so much vigour fifteen years after his death, and twenty-five years after it began.

Enid Balint
March 1986

Introduction

The general practice setting allows easy access to ten minutes of the doctor's time. Patients come to their doctors with a great variety of different kinds of distress. Frequently the emotional and physical aspects of illness occur together and intimately reflect each other. Doctors have been trained in medical school to 'do something' and often play this role on occasions when 'being someone' for their patients may be more helpful.

In vocational training for general practice nowadays emphasis is often laid on a general style of personal accessibility in consulting. Techniques are taught with the help of audio and video recordings of consultations. Although a doctor's outward manner may be modified by this sort of behavioural feedback, what use can he make of his more personal world for understanding his patients better? The 'video' is also needed in the doctor's head as a third eye, monitoring his reactions and feelings in response to the patient. This can then allow him to make freer and fuller use of his own personality in his professional work; a freeing from within his range of personal reactions rather than an imitative addition from without. The purpose of our work (and the reason for this book) is to promote a better understanding of what goes on between patients and those doctors trying to work in this way.

General practice has now emerged as a respected academic discipline from the dark depression that encompassed it when Michael and Enid Balint started working with general practitioners in the 1950s. Their ideas have now spread world-wide and consequently the training-research groups that they developed have been adapted in many ways. Essentially a Balint group still consists of about ten or twelve doctors who meet regularly every week for at least two years. The work consists entirely of case discussion, and usually only two or three patients are considered in a session of an hour and a half. Every doctor has patients that trouble him, and studying them carefully with colleagues helps him learn about his blind spots and how he might usefully modify his approach. The leader of the group is traditionally a psychoanalyst, but nowadays there are others who do this work after suitable training and experience. The task of the leader is to keep the group focused on the relationship between the doctor and patient. The leaders are not there to offer treatment to the doctor, nor to undermine his traditional medical role, but to help him understand how he is responding to patients. Inevitably such a learning process has its painful moments. For example a doctor may realize that he has been more concerned to please a patient than to help him, or that there are certain kinds of patients with whom he has special difficulties. The group needs to have continuity and a sense of involvement to allow its members time to develop their personal skills. Some groups meet, as did ours, to look beyond personal professional development and undertake research into particular aspects of general practice.

The work described here began in 1980, when we were invited by Enid Balint to join her in a project that was loosely defined as 'taking another look at the "Flash" ' – a concept which had arisen from the work of the group who wrote *Six Minutes for the Patient* in 1973. They had examined effective work based on understandings derived from Balint training, but carried out within the context of the normal short general practice consultation. In the course of that research, a number of interviews had been reported where there had been a sudden, even dramatic, moment of deepened understanding between doctor and patient, arising from the doctor's 'tuning in' to the patient's communication, rather than as a consequence of a deliberately directed enquiry or series of questions.

The members of our group had all had several years of Balint group experience and two had been members of the 'Six Minutes' group. The method was to be the usual Balint-style discussion of current cases, with recording and transcription of the meetings, to provide material that could be referred to later.

At our first meeting, problems of defining the 'Flash' were at once apparent and one doctor quoted an incident to see whether it fitted the picture. He recalled a consultation about three months before when, at the end of a long surgery, a rather mousy-looking girl in her late twenties had come in and said, 'It's my constipation doctor.' The doctor had already discussed this symptom with her on frequent previous attendances over several months, dutifully inquiring about her diet and advising modifications. Now, tired and fed up at the end of the evening, he groaned and said, 'No, not more constipation – I don't believe you have come to tell me about constipation.'

Suddenly the girl burst into tears. She then began to pour out a story of unrequited love and unhappiness and her inability to deal with it.

With this now in the open for the first time, the doctor and patient were able to have a long talk about the major problems in her life and her response to them. He had not seen her again since then.

We wondered what had caused the doctor to make this rather unprofessional comment. Was it purely an unguarded moment of exasperation or had there been something about this particular patient, that had elicited his response? The doctor was not consciously aware of having responded to any signal.

'I felt I'm not going to use my brain to understand you. I am too tired. I remember sitting there and feeling extremely despondent rather than being an intellectual doctor and listening and wondering, what does she mean by that?'

This tentatively offered case, which was not subsequently followed up because it preceded the real start of the group's work, now seems significant because it anticipated several matters which were to occupy our attention as the study progressed and are discussed in detail in later chapters of this book. One of these was the 'moment of change' itself – the unexpected shift of pace or direction within the consultation. Another was the way in which the doctor may drop his defences, taking a chance by behaving in a more personal rather than professional manner and finding that this enables the patient to do the same. The third pointer to the future work of the group was the problem of assessing outcome. This patient had attended six or seven times in five months with her symptom of constipation. Since the interview with its change of focus, she had not reappeared in three months. Did this represent an improvement, or did she not return because she was too frightened by the kind of 'medicine' she had received? What future use might the patient, or the doctor, make of this altered relationship between them?

There is a fundamental problem that besets those who attempt what has been called 'narrative research'. Clinical research has a clear sequence of events: define the problem, devise methods for studying it, and do a pilot study; then revise the method, collect the results, analyse the findings, and perhaps publish the answers. Some of the previous research done by Balint groups dealt with such specific topics as night calls, repeat prescriptions, requests for abortion, and so on. These matters allowed fairly precise definition and some of the conclusions could even be expressed numerically as well as in descriptive terms. However, it is often the case that what is of most interest is very hard to measure. Whenever we considered how to define the changes we were studying, we met this problem. If we felt an important moment had occurred that changed things between a doctor and a patient, how could we demonstrate its validity? How could we define the change and relate it to the important moment? There were too many uncertainties to attempt validating our work by making and ascertaining the accuracy of predictions. Instead, our approach had to be that of the natural historian; to attempt honest descriptive work and hope that by examining it we could come to some useful conclusions.

Our work mainly focused on consultations which had one common factor: that a significant moment occurred which altered the doctor's view of his patient, or the problem, in a way that might make some observable change in the subsequent doctor–patient relationship. Our aim was not simply to describe an incident which might enliven a consultation, the 'important moment' being not so significant in itself, but to try to examine the *content* of one interview within the *context* of the whole relationship.

It is very much our hope that all those who are involved with general practice through teaching or learning, as patients or practitioners, will find the description of our encounters with patients both interesting and helpful.

1
Uses and abuses of the consultation

Jack Norell

The general practice consultation with its long tradition has recently attracted the interest of two diametrically opposed schools. On the one side, the more holistic-than-thou, anything-goes, patients-know-as-much-as-doctors, sentimental wets; on the other, the precise, scientifically objective, myopic, technocratic, checklist-classifying behaviourists. The severe limitations of both these approaches are already becoming apparent, but we would do well to re-examine the nature of the time-honoured consultation. Does it do its job properly? Is it being employed effectively and efficiently? And what is its job in the first place? The purpose of this opening chapter is to review these questions.

For general practitioners, the consultation has a far greater significance than it does for colleagues in most other medical disciplines. The brief repeated encounters we have with our patients over the years represent virtually our sole arena, where almost everything we do as doctors is done. Practically all we achieve, we do there and then, 'while I'm here, doctor'.

In current jargon, general practice is regarded as low-technology and labour-intensive. Despite the inevitable dilution from sharing work with colleagues and staff, we offer continuity and remain personal. The past years have seen widespread attempts to improve our consulting, but in striving to do better we have possibly been trying too hard. The subject of consultation techniques has been opened up to the new sciences. Sociologists, educationalists, and psychologists with ideas about the importance of their theories have not been slow to proffer their assistance, eager to redefine the nature of general practice and to rewrite our approach to it (Pendleton *et al.* 1984). Jargon fills the atmosphere, and 'rules' abound. The field is littered with helpful guidance on interview techniques such as how the consulting room furniture ought to be arranged, where to sit, how to greet patients, when to respond, what to say, how to phrase it, where to look, and so on (Martin and Moulds 1986). Whether these particular styles of interviewing make the slightest difference to the eventual outcome of the consultation may be disputed, but they are deemed to be 'good things'. They conform to prevailing educational theory and are in keeping with the received wisdom of social psychologists. Above all, these techniques can be taught – and that justifies everything.

It may seem curious that so much emphasis should be placed on the way the consultation is structured and on its process, rather than looking at the eventual outcome. But this trend pervades the whole of general practice at present. Attention is focused on performing, on ways of doing things, on the process of caring, to the virtual exclusion of observing long-term results. There is an obvious reason for this. Conventional medical measures are either too crude (for example, mortality rates), or are simply not appropriate for general practice ('cure' rates for example). By the very nature of our work, long follow-up periods are necessary to reach any rational conclusions.

In this respect few general practice studies can match those emanating from Balint seminars, beginning with the original *The Doctor, his Patient, and the Illness* (Balint 1957), and including *Treatment or Diagnosis* (Balint *et al.* 1970), and *Six Minutes for the Patient* (Balint and Norell 1973). Comparing the results of different approaches by looking at outcomes is a necessary discipline, not so much because it is 'scientific', but because it is part and parcel of any profession's behaviour. If, as is often the case, it is found that a variety of different techniques give comparable results, then this raises the possibility that the condition being studied is self-limiting, that the procedures adopted may not be particularly relevant, or that the various techniques may be ritualistic rather than 'routine'.

Soliciting patients' accounts of the consultation may be a perfectly valid way of performing an external reality check. Although patients are rarely in a position to have a total view of what went on, they nevertheless must be the final arbiters on such things as how the doctor came over, how they felt they were being treated, whether they believed that they were being taken seriously. In this area, at least, the consumer is (very nearly) always right.

In the accounts of consultations quoted in this book, what comes over strikingly is the wide variety of styles, approaches, and techniques adopted by the doctors in our group. Clearly, the individual doctors were not afraid to be themselves. This freedom to be 'natural' did not come easily. Almost all Balint-trained doctors were originally much exercised over the 'right' thing to say, the 'appropriate' response, the 'correct' interpretation. Yet, looking at the way some of the reported consultations went, it does seem that what was important to patients was not so much what was actually said to them, as how they were treated. Words of course play a part in the latter, but there is much else besides.

The patient's perception of how things went during the consultation may not match the doctor's. A number of studies (notably those of Ann Cartwright in 1966 and 1981) have revealed interesting discrepancies. Evidently it is not enough that the doctor should be concerned, attentive, and caring. Like justice, these things must be seen to be done. For instance, going through the motions of an otherwise unimportant physical examination is often of value for patients; the act of touching being important in itself.

Often the doctor can 'tell at a glance' what the matter is and decide rapidly what is required. But there are occasions when swift judgement and the subsequent short cuts may be counterproductive. Sometimes the long journey has to be undertaken, doctor and patient together, painfully slowly if necessary, but in any event never faster than the patient.

It appears then, that a variety of styles of consulting are compatible with 'good doctoring'. The doctor may be courageous or cautious, openly active or apparently passive, probing or minimally responsive. These techniques do not themselves obviously influence the final result. What does matter is that the doctor be perceptive, shrewd, imaginative, and thoughtful. Above all, experience counts, provided having 'heard it all before' does not make the doctor feel jaded and so rob the encounter of its sense of newness. An important attribute for doctors engaged in this kind of work is the capacity to retain interest – even better, curiosity – about patients and their lives. A little naïveté on the part of the doctor can sometimes work wonders.

All doctors, other than out-and-out behaviourists, would agree that an important step for them is to obtain insight into the patient's situation. (Whether patients themselves need insight before they can be helped is another matter.) For general practitioners, the necessary insight extends beyond mere knowledge of the facts. It also falls short of the very ambitious aim of achieving an understanding of the whole patient. In our gradually evolving relationship with patients we are mostly offered only glimpses of moving fragments from which we are expected to discern the wider scene; a tough assignment indeed.

Is a full understanding of the comprehensive picture really necessary, even if it were possible? Perhaps not, for the approach of really experienced general practitioners relies more on selectivity than on omniscience. The extent and depth of insight required by the doctor should be sufficient to enable him to sense what it must be like to be that patient. This acquisition is crucial and its absence is at the root of many of our difficulties with troubled and troublesome patients.

Without this level of insight, relationships may remain superficial or unproductive, leading to doctor and patient being at cross purposes. When the doctor reflects to himself, 'if I were him . . .', in truth he is really picturing, 'if he were me . . .'.

It has been observed that to obtain a true understanding requires one to 'stand under'. A sense of humility is called for, a deference to the real expert – the patient. Further, 'shared understanding' implies a total congruence of the doctor's and patient's respective notions. But as some of the quoted consultations illustrate, a patient may later say something which reveals them both to be poles apart. It is more realistic to recognize the shifting nature of such 'understandings' and to be grateful for those fleeting moments when doctor and patient appear to be on the same wave-length.

These moments were often associated with the doctor's observation of something incongruous or even frankly preposterous in the patient's presentation. Occasionally, it was preceded by negative feelings on the part of the doctor: disdain, disapproval, dislike, scorn, or contempt. It is interesting that such feelings, however undesirable they may seem, can sometimes actually have a productive effect on the consultation and assist the development of the relationship. In this sense, these 'unacceptable' feelings have a far less numbing effect on the consultation than fear of the patient or hatred, which can virtually sterilize the doctor–patient encounter.

Possibly, too much attention has been paid to the 'flash' itself. It has been treated as a source of wonder, just as lightning itself tends to be. We ought instead to be noting its practical effect in 'lighting up' the scene, illuminating momentarily that which was previously in comparative darkness. At present we do not know how to make it happen, but we should accept that it does happen without warning and resolve to make good use of it when it does.

The conduct of the consultation has to be seen against the wider aims of general practice which go beyond the traditional concept of 'medical care', as understood in our hospitals for instance. We now accept that our role is not just to restore people to their former condition, where this is possible, but to conserve their health by suitable preventive measures, and to try to promote it by advice and education, these strategies being dignified by the terms curative medicine, preventive medicine, and health education respectively.

Nowadays we are much less enamoured of our curative role than we were, recognizing the inherent limitations of being general practitioners. Nevertheless, our image is still of someone who 'makes people better'. This doctor is not expected to initiate any moves but to wait until his advice is sought 'by a person who is ill or who believes himself to be ill' (Spence 1960), whereupon he springs into action. This stance resembles that of the spider, poised motionless until triggered into activity.

Things are changing. Increasingly in our conventional medical work we take the initiative in such matters as child surveillance, immunization, cervical smears, screening for hypertension, and so on. In doing so we are adopting the principles of preventive medicine and helping to 'keep people better'. At the same time there is more emphasis on health education, with advice on eating, smoking, and drinking for example; because we realize that many ills can be regarded today as partly self-inflicted and that we are moving into a realm where public health measures are largely ineffective and only the patient's own decisions can have any impact.

There is not a great enthusiasm among us for the concept of positive mental health, or 'complete mental well-being'. Our reticence is probably well-founded for we know little enough about the prerequisites for assisting people to reach their full potential in this area and may not feel justified in intervening with gratuitous advice, whether of the positive or negative kind.

Instead, we prefer to wait to be consulted by patients who are sufficiently troubled to seek outside help, whose threshold of tolerance has been exceeded, or who have literally been made ill by their personal problems. This can be a perfectly legitimate professional posture and in the present state of the art it is probably the safest, wisest, and most practicable approach. But this stance carries a number of important conditions to do with the doctor's accessibility, sensitivity, and awareness.

If the onus is wholly on the patient to initiate a consultation on matters which have a significant emotional component, then the doctor's personal availability becomes crucial. This implies more than actually getting to see the doctor – it means getting through to him as well. In turn, this has implications for the doctor's sensibility: his sensitivity to what patients are trying to express (and trying not to), and his self-awareness about conscious and barely conscious constraints and conditions he imposes on patients. For instance, the sort of illness ('ticket of entry') they are entitled to present with and how distressed they have to be in the first place. Doctors have their own thresholds for 'hearing' and for agreeing to get involved in exploring patients' personal problems.

Fewer Balint-trained doctors today pursue deliberate, systematic psychotherapy of the classical sort with their patients. Many did become quite skilled at it but there was always an aura of 'Sunday best' about the way it was reserved for special patients on special occasions.

How to incorporate those hard-won skills into our daily activities was the task for the second phase of the Balint movement. Shortage of time is repeatedly offered as the reason why 'busy general practitioners' cannot adopt the lessons which have emerged from the Balint approach. But as Enid Balint has observed, in this sort of work achievements in the consultation are not time-related but intensity-related. Beyond this there was the hope that this approach could be thoroughly integrated into our ordinary work and used as the opportunity presented itself during our unplanned and unstructured consultations. Indeed, we have succeeded in making a virtue out of necessity; opportunism in general practice has always been respectable.

A more realistic perspective was placed on our traditional 'curative' role by the classical injunction, 'to cure sometimes, relieve often, comfort always'. The word 'comfort' is commonly understood to mean 'soothing', but in fact its root clearly indicates its association with giving strength (just as 'encouraging' means 'giving heart'). Real comfort should confer on the patient the ability to cope with his problem – independently of the doctor eventually. Comfort is greatly superior to mere support, for it conveys to the patient the equivalent of 'pull yourself together'; which is to say, 'I am concerned for you; you are worth bothering about; you have it in you to get over this.'

An ideal system of health care would cater for all manifestations of ailing, patients being allowed to be ill in the way most natural to them. The various psychotherapeutic approaches to states of 'dis-ease' were supposed to liberate the patient from the need to fit into the traditional medical classification of bodily and mental disorders. But Procrustes is alive and well and he thrives in precisely those allegedly enlightened circles which proclaim 'non-directive' and 'non-judgemental' attitudes. Patients are still being fitted into theories of behaviour and notions of game-playing. They are still labelled and classified not nowadays by one-word diagnoses, but in paragraphs of 'formulation'.

The general practitioner does of course have cases of hypochondriasis and neurosis, but it is interesting how their numbers seem to diminish as the doctor gets to know his patients. Not that their outward behaviour is any less demanding or aggressive, but the doctor can see that there is considerably more to them than that. Conventional diagnostic terms then seem inappropriate; and even a comprehensive formulation may not adequately capture the significant features of the unique individual.

Doctors may pursue their aims in a bewildering variety of ways. Some engage in active exploration; delving, probing, nudging, prodding, or otherwise stimulating patients to voice their thoughts and – especially – their feelings. They are busy leaving no stone unturned, no emotion unexpressed. Other doctors seem content to wait for the patient to make the moves and confine themselves to signalling their availability, interest, and willingness to be involved. In between are the many permutations of approach.

To a very large extent these differences reflect doctors' personalities rather than the way they were trained. Some seem to wear the label 'caring doctor' and openly brandish their compassion. Others are more reserved, guarded, or neutral. Each runs the risk of being regarded as either intrusive or uncaring. Similar differences attend the way the patient's statement is treated. If the doctor takes it at its face value, he may be thought of as naïve. If he speculates on its 'real' meaning he may be accused of reading into it much more than it warrants. The doctor's imagination is an important part of his armamentarium but needs to be applied with discretion. If there were such a thing as disciplined fantasizing, then that might be the real recipe.

Enthusiasm is a marvellous attribute and should never have cold water poured on it. It is one of the most significant ingredients in the provision of decent care for patients, but it needs cultivating so that it does not get out of hand. Otherwise we may see the doctor taking off and leaving his patient some way behind, raising the suspicion that the doctor is on some sort of ego trip and has not properly curbed his need to be needed. (There is the story of the boy scout, determined to do his good deed that day, who propelled an elderly lady to the other side of a road she had not intended to cross.)

It is undoubtedly true that some of our 'captive' patients are being harassed in subtle and not so subtle ways. Patients who do not 'realize' what their problem is – or even that they have a problem – are being 'helped' to achieve a proper understanding; that is, their doctor's understanding. Whose problem is actually being addressed during such exercises? Doctors are shutting patients up with interpretations, pre-empting discussion, and rail-roading them into promising areas; paying only lip-service to the need for continual negotiation with the patient on what the focus of attention should be.

We hear less nowadays of the arrogant term 'problem-solving techniques' applied to consultations in general practice. Problem-defining, perhaps, though even this may be too ambitious at times, when all one can hope for is to explore in the hope of discovering not *the* problem but a new light on several related problems.

The purpose of defining problems is to arrive at solutions. Here again the doctor experiences a dilemma. Respect for the patient's autonomy means recognizing that the patient is ultimately responsible for his own salvation. But how can a member of a caring, helping profession stand by while 'false' solutions are being adopted by his patient? It is this prospect which makes many of us take a protective stance towards our patients. Not to do so would be abdicating a responsibility, while doing so might be seen as arrogating one. Truly, we cannot win. We rightly encourage self-help, but might there still be a place for 'doctor's orders'? Are there not some patients in need of paternalism at times? Is it possible to have this without being patronized?

Another potential source of conflict for the doctor is the concept of an agenda for the consultation. Since the patient normally initiates the encounter he may be considered the appropriate person to write the agenda for it. The doctor may also have legitimate items to include, things to do with preventive medicine for instance, or other matters which shout out for attention but which the patient ignores. It is for each doctor to decide how far these items represent a 'retreat' into conventional health care and an avoidance of persevering with the more difficult exploration of the patient's own territory. He also has to decide where, in his own set of professional values, he places waiting and watchfulness – an implicit part of the pastoral approach – compared to the need for patient compliance.

More damaging, possibly, than open conflict is the collusion which creates a gentleman's agreement not to trespass into certain areas. Encouragement to intrude into such sensitive places is an inevitable part of any doctor's training process and often brings forth the familiar penalties of scolding and rapped knuckles. Furthermore, being warned off in such an unmistakable way can turn out to be a misleading experience for the doctor because the same patient at a later date may recognize the need for that exploratory approach and actually seek it.

The traditional medical posture towards emotional matters was characterized by a deliberate distancing, a no-touch technique. Patients' feelings were regarded as distractions which contaminated the 'real' medical issues. As for doctors' feelings, these were totally beyond the pale and their existence strenuously denied. In redressing this constraining attitude it was inevitable that the pendulum should swing too far in the opposite direction, so that closeness, proximity, intimacy, and the free expression of feelings should be regarded as the key to successful doctor–patient relationships.

Perhaps being scorched is not a bad way of discovering that there is such a thing as 'too close for comfort'. At all events, experienced doctors are well aware of the concept of optimal distance which varies from patient to patient and, more bafflingly, for the same patient from time to time. Despite this distance, or perhaps because of it, it is still possible to convey proper professional concern and respect for the person.

A more searching test of the quality of the doctor–patient relationship would be its degree of honesty. Again, total openness and honesty are not common features of doctor–patient relationships (any more than of other relationships) and we must look for more realistic criteria. One which is significant and highly relevant to the way our work seems to be evolving relates to the concept of the patient's use of the doctor. Being 'used' has a derogatory connotation, yet when the horror has receded it is possible to appreciate its appropriateness, and indeed to admire its logic. It entails a total shift from our profession's previous haughty reliance (and nagging insistence) on 'patient compliance', and recognizes that in one sense the patient does ultimately call the tune – whether or not he directly pays the piper.

A widely accepted job description of general practice includes the statement that the doctor shall reach a decision on any problem presented to him by his patient. Often enough, that decision may be 'not to get involved' and there are many ways open to general practitioners to avoid engaging with troubled patients. (Our specialist colleagues also have their alibis, such as describing patients as unco-operative, non-compliant, poorly motivated, or resistant.) It is sometimes difficult to remember that the important thing for the patient is the opportunity to have his say, to present his case, however falteringly. It is in creating an atmosphere in which the patient can feel secure enough to do this that the doctor makes a major contribution to a worthwhile consultation.

An ancient description of the doctor credited him with being guide, philosopher, and friend. It can scarcely be bettered as an overall view of the field of work of the general practitioner, reflecting as it does his multi-faceted role in the consultation. First and foremost (in the patient's eyes, certainly) the doctor gives guidance on medical matters. He is not a provider, prescriber, administrator, or organizer, but a medical adviser. In helping patients to be 'philosophical' he conveys, but does not impose, a sense of values. As Michael Balint was fond of pointing out, the doctor is a teacher who brings to patients an understanding of, among other things, what has to be borne, what (however unfashionable today) must be endured (Balint 1957). What the patient wants of his doctor is to be befriended; and a true friend means being a candid friend.

With the adoption of psychoanalysis as a model for the kind of psychotherapeutic work general practitioners tended to engage in, there grew the belief that the last thing the doctor must do was to allow his feelings to show. But impassivity and inscrutability are not particularly appropriate poses for the general practitioner who is also friend to his patients and this style can often baffle and even frighten them. By contrast, the doctor who decides for instance not to conceal his disappointment or disapproval may in fact be helping to develop a more productive relationship than if he were to assume the outward appearance of tolerance while fuming inwardly.

One test of a good relationship is that it can survive candour – from either of the two parties. Being natural is probably safer than many doctors imagine. Patients are more tolerant and adaptable to doctors' styles than we give them credit for. In any case, the intuitive response can often be superior to the painfully laboured, contrived, self-conscious effort of the 'trained' doctor.

Another common fallacy is the high value attached to precision and explicitness by the doctor in the interest of 'good communication'. It is possible to overburden patients with facts and to confuse them by 'explanations'. Apart from this, there may be positive value in the doctor's being vague, tentative, speculative, or even ambiguous. If asked by the patient to explain what he means, the doctor's slowness to do so may not necessarily be evasive. He may genuinely not be sure what he 'really' means. Meanwhile, through an association of ideas the patient may have been able to use the doctor's comment to bring other ideas forward.

Reassurance, much sought after by nearly all patients, has acquired a rather contemptible reputation among Balint-trained doctors, but it does have a legitimate place in the consultation. There is an important proviso however; the doctor must first accurately identify the source of the patient's worry, or at least uncover the accompanying circumstances. Only when the specific concern – however irrational – has been elicited can proper reassurance be given. In other words, 'diagnosis first, treatment afterwards'. There is as little place for jovial, back-slapping, blanket reassurance as there is for blunderbuss therapy of other kinds.

Balint-trained doctors were among the first to reverse the familiar aphorism, converting it to 'don't just do something, sit there!'. But the value of the doctor's 'being there' was greatly underrated originally. Doctors constantly strove to say the right things, make the right noises, give the right response and this is still a preoccupation for some of us. The craze for 'telling' apparently knows no bounds and no doubt reflects the touching belief that patients can be talked out of their worries. An example of this is one counselling technique, said to be appropriate for general practice, which involves searching for any 'irrational beliefs' that might be upsetting the patient (such as the awfulness of their spouses, or how useless they feel themselves to be) and then disputing these mistakenly held ideas. Successful disputation by the doctor, it is alleged, leads to a change from irrational to rational belief, and thus to a change in behaviour and feelings (Tutton and Dryden 1983). Reminiscent, no doubt, of 'every day, in every way . . .'

Nevertheless, it is not the mere presence of the doctor that works the oracle. (Admittedly it may seem like this sometimes when, for instance, the doctor is preoccupied with other thoughts or switched off for any number of reasons, and yet the patient carries on as if inspired.) What really counts for the patient is the evidence that he matters; that his doctor is giving attention and not just listening but *hearing*. That there is someone responsible available, not to do or say anything particularly, but available. The message for us doctors is clear. Understand your patients if you can; love them if you must; but for Heaven's sake, notice them.

2
Fact or fiction?

John Salinsky

How do Balint-trained doctors actually work? There seems to be a number of popular misconceptions around. If you were to ask the average doctor in his surgery what he thought about Balint work, he might say something like this:

'I read the Balint book when I was a trainee. Very interesting of course, but not very practical, is it? Some doctors get very keen on it and get together in groups, but you can only do that in London. They tend to believe that when a patient comes in time after time with trivial complaints it's really because he has a sex problem and a Balint doctor will do his best to get to the bottom of it. He will bring the patient back out of surgery hours and have long sessions delving into his childhood and all that sort of thing. They claim that it saves time in the end because the patients stop coming back with aches and pains and sore throats once the doctor has shown them what's *really* wrong with them; but I don't believe it myself. Mind you, I'm not saying it's a lot of rubbish. In fact I use Balint myself from time to time, but only when it's appropriate. These days there are so many other behavioural techniques you can use, or you can send them to a counsellor or a psychologist.'

This is admittedly something of a caricature. The Balint doctor is seen as taking a firm grip of a patient with tedious physical symptoms and applying a specialized technique of psychiatric enquiry to elicit a psychological, preferably sexual, diagnosis. The correct interpretation is then expected to produce an instant cure. No wonder the average general practitioner is sceptical. The experience of being in a Balint group is very different; less sensational and more recognizably to do with ordinary doctoring. Here is the first of three cases reported to our group. The cases are described by using edited material from the transcript of the doctor's report.

ALISON

She is a girl who is quite small, sort of untidy with stringy hair and a bit of a mess. She's got two kids. She looks about 18 or 19, but in fact she's 31. I have seen her three times before. She first came my way last April complaining of being tired and having painful periods and being generally worried about herself and her marriage. It was all sort of mushy unhappy stuff. I saw her again a couple of weeks later when she was complaining much more about the physical symptoms, about the aches and pains and that it was impossible to have sex because it hurt so much and she was in tears and was depressed and she had to work and her job was important to her and was difficult. I was uncertain at the time whether she was physically ill or emotionally upset or what the hell. I took some blood for a test and gave her some Mianserin (an antidepressant), hedging my bets both ways. And she came back a couple of weeks later feeling rather better, but she hadn't taken the pills because the first one upset her. I advised her to come back in a month and she turned up this week, that is eight months later. It was a Monday morning, things were a bit harassed and we were running late. The whole interview lasted about ten minutes. She complained of sore eyes and I advised her to give up smoking. I got the feeling that I was giving her platitudes and she was responding with appropriate irritation. So I just shut up for a bit and she then started talking about how angry she felt. Her husband sits and plays with his home computer in the evenings; she said, 'I'm quite happy about that, but the real trouble is I keep on having outbursts of temper. I lose my temper and I hate the kids and I scream at my husband and I really don't mean it. My husband is a gentle soul, he worries about me being unhappy and it's just not fair. There's been no sex for five months and I don't enjoy it.'

The whole thing was depressive and I was thinking Oh my God, one miserable girl who can't do a damn thing for anybody. I got a feeling that she was launching at me but she didn't want me to do anything about it. So I said something about she sounded as if she was feeling very insecure and unhappy and she was pretty ashamed of being as useless as this. And that was the thing that really seemed to be helpful because she started talking about the nice things of her job. She is a purchasing officer and she can be competent there and quite good and she comes home and she could be competent as a housewife, but then her husband and the children are dependent on her and she really resents people relying on her. She said, 'I have to stifle that, I can't own up to them.' I got this feeling that while she resents being depended on she was at the same time acting in a very dependent way towards me and I pointed this out to her. I then said, 'You know you've told me a certain amount about yourself. What would you like now? What do you want from us? Would you like to come back?' She said: 'Look, I think we've been saying something that's helpful and I don't want to come back unless *I* want to. Can I go and think about it?' And I said, 'Sure, come back when you want to, if you want to.' And that was the end of the interview. It was a rather messy interview in which something seemed to have been useful.

What are we to make of this? It certainly isn't a long analysis in depth, we are told that it only lasted ten minutes. The doctor doesn't deploy any specialized technique: he simply perceives that he's being a bit pompous and decides to shut up and listen after which Alison feels free to pour out her frustrations. She doesn't like to feel that she has to be an emotional support for her family, and the doctor then points out that she is asking him to do the same for her. Instead of pressing on with further interpretations and perhaps endangering her need to feel independent, the doctor instead allows her to go away and think about whether she wants to come again and how she would like to use his help. There is no conclusion, no advice, no prescription, and no referral. There has, however, been a change in the relationship between doctor and patient. They have drawn closer and been more frank with one another. The doctor has greater warmth and respect for her, now seeing her in a more balanced way. She realizes that he has responded to something important about her.

In the group discussion which followed there was great interest in whether the patient would change as a result of this interview, whether she would come back to the doctor and in what sort of frame of mind.

In the second example a change in the quality of the relationship between patient and doctor was apparently touched off by the crash of some dishes accidentally falling to the floor.

EDNA
This lady is a widow I have known for twenty years. She is 76 years old now, I don't know how many times she's attended, but it's over a hundred in the years I've known her. Her daughter and grandson are also my patients. She rouses a lot of negative emotions in me; I have had phases of being terribly energetic and trying to get her rehoused, but mostly by now I'm frustrated and exasperated and rather dread her turning up. She suffers from quite bad, genuine rheumatoid arthritis. She's had endless problems with a repair. Her most recent complaint has been hypertension and she comes in regularly for tablets and to have her blood pressure taken. Ten days ago she came in I can't remember why and I was feeling a bit irritated. Because I really feel I

have done all I possibly can, we never seem to be further on and she sits there looking terribly miserable and exhausted. I think she was giddy this morning, but she's been giddy quite a lot recently and we adjust her tablets and she's a little less giddy or a little more giddy, but it never makes any difference in the end.

Oh yes, she thought she had got some wax in her ear and I went over to my little table to get the auroscope and I was feeling a bit grotty and several things fell over. My irritation was obvious. And she giggled! She suddenly looked much younger – much more like her daughter. I commented on this in some way and she started telling me all about the war when the children were evacuated and she was a cleaner at the old East End Maternity Hospital and lots of amusing things had happened. I tried many years ago when I was stuck on long interviews to sort her out on more than one occasion with no success at all and I've never managed to get her to talk about her past. It was the first time in twenty years and over a hundred interviews that she ever really talked about anything other than her symptoms. When the children were evacuated they went down to Bournemouth to stay with a clergyman for a bit and a doctor for a bit and she was sure that was why Kathleen had such nice manners. She went on for about twenty minutes or so and I don't think she even had a prescription. And she went. I haven't seen her since. But it was quite a different interview to those I have had with her before. It seemed to be precipitated by me knocking over a pile of kidney dishes!

This began as yet another in a long line of tedious frustrating consultations. The doctor felt she had tried everything including trying to be a 'Balint doctor' and having long interviews. Nothing had made any difference to the patient's moaning and misery. Suddenly the dishes go over, the doctor is off balance, the patient giggles, looks younger, and the situation is used to strike a more human note with each other. The patient starts talking about herself in an entirely new way and the doctor listens with a renewed interest. In the group discussion the doctor was asked about the various strategies she had tried in the past to 'get through' to Edna. The doctor replied that even when her work had been 'clinically correct' and helpful, it didn't give the patient 'any joy whatever'. Now, she said, 'I feel "that's interesting", I'm looking forward to the next time she comes.' The group wondered whether Edna now had a different view of her doctor and how this might be utilized. Some people felt that it was better not to try too hard. The doctor should be content with the feeling that the next twenty years with Edna might be easier to bear.

MICHAEL

Michael is aged 48 and he is a very soft-spoken Irish man, quiet, sort of middle height, with greyish hair, glasses, rather insignificant. I had not seen him before. I just had a card. I was under some pressure so that I wasn't looking for anything that was going to go on for a long time. He came out straight away by saying that he had had claustrophobia for about ten years and he wanted a letter to go somewhere for treatment. It had started after an experience ten years ago in a tube train when the train was stopped for an hour and over the next few weeks he found increasing difficulty in travelling on various forms of transport. He couldn't go in the back of a car that didn't have rear doors. He flies on holiday once a year, sort of premedicated with Librium. I had a feeling about him at that point that he might be homosexual, but I asked how is the family, and he's got a wife and grown-up son. He mentioned hypnotherapy and I said well, that was a possibility, but I thought perhaps something along behavioural lines might be more useful and I mentioned the Maudsley. I was going to write him a letter and he said well I see you are busy. I'll pick up the letter in a day or two. Which quite surprised me because my patients aren't usually so considerate. They don't usually think of that sort of thing. So I said if you'd like to ring the Maudsley and see if they'll accept you. He came in again a week later and reported that the hospital wouldn't be able to offer him treatment for several months, but somebody might see him in the meantime. I usually write my letters in longhand while the patient is waiting. I thought I'd better write a bit more detail so I started asking a little bit more about his experiences. How had it happened? And he told me a bit more about the initial episode when he was in a very crowded train which stopped for a long time in a tunnel. It got more and more hot and he began to feel a bit faint. He was afraid of losing control of himself. There was a woman there who in a sense did lose control; she got very agitated, took her shoe off, and started hammering on the windows and that obviously made quite an impression on him. I said to him, 'why is it so important that you shouldn't lose control?' He gave me some rather bland answers. And then I said, 'why do you think I asked you that question?' He said, 'well, you are thinking . . . who do I think I am? Am I so important that it matters if I lose control?' That somehow fascinated me; that he should have thought I was kind of getting at him. I said I wasn't meaning to be so critical. I had just wondered what it meant to him. He said that when he was quite young, he was afraid of fainting and I had a picture of a large Irish family going to Mass on Sunday morning having had no breakfast. Quite frequently he would feel faint and felt it was terribly important that he shouldn't faint and lose control. He really hung on to himself so that he wouldn't actually pass out in church. I had more or less written my letter, but we'd stopped in the middle while that particular transaction came up. And I said to him, 'well, I think I'll have this letter typed, it will look better and I'll send it and ask them to send you an appointment.'

And then he said, 'well, um, if you've got time, there are one or two other things.' So he said did I think it was okay if he started jogging. So I took his blood pressure and that was all right, so I said it would be okay if he started jogging, if he took it gradually. And then he said, 'there's one other thing, but perhaps it would be better . . . would you rather I saw one of the male doctors about it?' So I said, 'well, what is it?' And he said that he had a swelling in his testis. I said, 'well, let's have a look.' I examined him and he had a slight thickening of the epididymis which might have been a small cyst but didn't seem anything of great significance so I said, 'I'll leave that for the moment and I'll look at it again in two or three weeks.' And that was really the end of the interview. The whole thing only lasted about ten minutes.

If we trace the events of the second interview we find the doctor initially asking one or two questions merely to amplify her letter of referral. Then she is struck first by his fear of losing control and then by his feeling that he is very insignificant and of no consequence to her. He has begun to come into focus as a real person who can feel hurt. The patient seems to be aware of the doctor's increased receptivity and is able to talk quite freely about his childhood. He decides that it is worth telling her about some physical worries and reveals some anxiety about his genitals.

There was general agreement that the doctor had become more interested and the patient more trusting – and perhaps that was as far as one could go. Perhaps the Balint Doctor of popular mythology would by this time have seized on the 'real' problem and got down to a searching examination of the patient's sexual fantasies. This doctor, on the other hand, was content to have established a relationship in which this apprehensive, self-deprecating patient can feel more free to talk.

What do these three stories tell us about the three doctors and their style of work? Are they using a specialized technique which enables them to look beyond each patient's 'trivial complaints' and interpret him to himself? It doesn't look like it. All three doctors seem to have felt fairly helpless and adrift at the beginning of the consultations. Then after a while, just when everything seems hopeless, something happens to make the doctor wake up and become more interested, not so much in the patient's pathology, but in the experience of being with him and listening to him. It seems to be the patients rather than the doctor who bring about the change, although they are probably unaware of doing so. Alison says: I'm not just a pathetic drudge; I'm really quite good at my job. Edna is jolted by the crash of the falling dishes and the doctor's dignity: she seems to shed forty years and become the more lively person she was in the blitz. Michael says (indirectly): I am afraid that I'm not important enough to matter to you – and then, for a while, he does.

After one of these turning points or 'important moments', the relationship seems to become more intimate and engaged where it had previously been distant and formal. The doctor feels that the patient has become likeable, forgivable, and understandable. He begins to believe that some progress is possible (Alison), or at least that the next twenty years with that patient will be more bearable (Edna). We know what the doctors experience because they have told us. But what is it like from the patients' viewpoint? How can we know whether anything has really changed for them? Has it been in any sense therapeutic? We need to know what happened in subsequent consultations.

ALISON

She did not appear again until two months later when she brought her 8-year-old son for treatment of his asthma. At the very end of the consultation her doctor said, 'How are things?' Alison said: 'Yes, fine,' and went on to say that after the previous interview it had been a help to be aware of the way she reacted, especially with her husband. 'She seemed,' said the doctor, 'to be the competent mother of her asthmatic son.'

Her next attendance was five weeks later. Again she brought her little boy and asked about the management of his asthma. When this had been dealt with, she asked him to wait outside and asked if she was due for a smear test (which she was). She complained of dysmenorrhoea and mittelschmerz. Things at home were much the same and they had sex rarely. She referred to our first discussion and said that she was afraid of talking about sex with her husband in case it made him feel 'on the spot'. The last time they had sex – five weeks ago – she had been left itching for weeks afterwards. She was given an appointment for a week later to take things further.

On the next visit she was examined vaginally and a smear was taken (she was relaxed and the routine procedure was completed without comment). She was looking smart and attractive and said that she was feeling much better. She had decided not to talk with her husband about their sex life and relationship. I said I felt that she didn't want to discuss the matter further with me either, but that if she wanted to look at the problem later with me, I would be happy to find time for this.

She said she felt very bad about taking up my time and then went on to tell me that she was very close with the wife of a local general practitioner who had been on my training course and that he thought very highly of me. I told her how much I liked him and the interview closed with warm mutual feelings of esteem and silent agreement to leave things as they were at the moment.

In this account it is striking that the patient describes herself as being 'very close with the wife of a local general practitioner'. It seems to suggest a fantasy just below the surface of consciousness that she *is* the wife of a local general practitioner, i.e. of her own doctor. How nice it would be, she imagines, to be as close to this sympathetic doctor as his wife. The doctor seems unaware of these unspoken thoughts or at any rate doesn't interpret them. But the interview closes 'with warm mutual feelings' and Alison seems to be happier for having been understood and accepted. There have been no long sessions, but somehow this understated relationship has itself been therapeutic. She has attended regularly and she seems to feel more peaceful. We don't know if anything will change at home.

The doctor's final report was that she had attended once more (with a sick child). Then, four months later, she came to ask if she and her family could remain as patients even though they were moving to a better house in another district. The doctor explained that this was not possible and she thanked him warmly for looking after them.

EDNA

There was a gap of five months and then, in the course of the next seven months, another eight consultations, each lasting five to ten minutes. Here is a sample, nearly a year after the initial reported interview:

She had wax in her ear and her knee was worse. She was seen together with a student. She came in smiling and was delighted to have a student examine her knee. She was friendly and chatty.

Two weeks later: she had fallen over her own feet, had pain in her right shoulder and her right knee. After an X-ray at hospital she had been told there was no bony injury. She laughed about this in a wry way. Her blood pressure is under control at present.

The doctor commented: 'I no longer find her such a burden. She's much more cheerful and forthcoming. Her visits are of the same frequency but shorter and chattier and much less trying. She seems to be prepared to show me different aspects of herself.'

MICHAEL

He came again two weeks later to have his testicle re-examined; there were two or three slightly hard areas in the epididymis, just as before, and I said I'd refer him to somebody about that. I thought I would take the opportunity, while he was getting dressed and I was washing my hands, to ask him whether it gave him any trouble when he had intercourse with his wife. I suppose I was trying to find out whether he did have intercourse with her. He just said, 'No, it's all right, you know.' And I think I asked twice. At the end I just sat down and wrote the letter for the surgical out-patients and that was it.

The group members were all rather disappointed that this patient had 'gone off the boil' and no longer felt the relaxed freedom to talk that he had experienced in the first interview. Had the doctor been wrong to enquire about his sexuality in this slightly oblique way? Had he been frightened off? There was speculation about how this fitted in with Michael's fear of losing control. The doctor felt that she had been both too tentative and too impatient; too much aware of the other group members' desire to hear more details. At the end of the discussion somebody said: 'Your understanding was really about religion, not about sex.'

In the following month Michael attended the Urology Clinic where he was found to have a small epididymal cyst. He attended the Maudsley Hospital where he was offered behaviour therapy, but declined to take it up. Nine months later he consulted his doctor's partner because his claustrophobia was worse. He was treated with desensitization and antidepressants at another hospital, was off work for several months but subsquently improved and returned to work, according to his wife whom the doctor sees occasionally. She (the doctor) had not seen Michael again and commented: 'He has seen several doctors in the practice and I don't think he has any particular allegiance. The initial encounter does not seem to have had any lasting significance.'

These follow-up reports seem to add up to one possible success, one modest improvement, and one failure. Not a very auspicious score when considered in this way, but I think such a superficial summary would be quite misleading. It is only the mythological 'Balint Doctor' who claims to 'cure' patients by interpreting their symptoms. The doctors in our group were not attempting anything of this kind. What they did was to encourage the development of a therapeutic relationship which the patient could then use as much or as little as he wanted. They were able to let this happen because they were interested in their patients' lives and in what they wanted from a visit to the doctor. This is quite different from making a conventional diagnosis (whether physical or psychological) and treating in the approved manner whether the patient wants it or not.

3
Search or serendipity?
Oliver Samuel

What has to happen to change a routine attendance at the doctor's surgery into something more significant? Do doctors deliberately choose patients to whom they respond with additional interest, or is it something that happens more spontaneously? The following account attempts to examine how the work begins.

There were some predictable openings. The doctor may know that the patient has, for example, been recently bereaved and offer his concern to see if the patient would welcome a friendly listening ear. A patient may make a conscious and deliberate decision to seek help. Sometimes patients have to struggle quite hard to find a gap in the doctor's routine. Occasionally, for no obvious reason, something just happens and both patient and doctor start working on a different plane.

Some of the cases reported to our group will be described in order to illustrate these situations. They are presented in the words of the doctor who had treated the patient. Only the beginnings of the cases are described so as to focus on the opening moments. What happened later is described in the Appendix.

MRS ISAACS

I saw an old lady in an old people's home today. I do a regular call there and I'd seen four or five people and at the end of the time this woman came to the door and said 'I'm sorry doctor, I didn't put my name down, but I wanted to see you.' I said 'Come in and sit down.' She's one who had come in since Christmas and I couldn't think exactly who she was. She's rather striking with full make-up and very soigné sort of blue-tinted hair. She's eighty or more and very neatly dressed. She'd had a fall and hurt her back, so I asked her what had happened. She had had a nightmare and fallen out of bed.

I really felt that this was an offer I shouldn't resist. But I was in difficulties because I couldn't remember exactly who she was. So when she said, 'my room is terrible, so poky, and shut in,' I was able to ask which room it was. A quick glimpse down my list of residents gave me her name at last and I was able to pay full attention and ask about her terrible dream. She said, 'Oh . . . I was trying to escape from this awful institution.' She comes from the Cotswolds and had a beautiful home. Her husband died, but she has two daughters who want to look after her, so she has come to this home to be near them. Suddenly she can't stand how it actually is; all drooling, senile, and depressed. She got onto this and shed a tear or two and I felt how awful it would be and was able to sort of share that with her.

Had the doctor known exactly who the patient was, then the change in the quality of the interview would hardly have been so dramatic. The patient seems to have been in need of a personal doctor to help prevent her from feeling senile and unwanted. The doctor couldn't even put a name to her and struggled more to learn who she was, than to find out what help she needed. The patient felt overwhelmed by the anonymous institutional atmosphere and the threat of losing her own faculties and dignity. Fortunately this turned out to be the key to the patient's nightmares. Both the doctor and the patient were actually experiencing in parallel very similar feelings about the loss of the patient's identity. Once he was able to put a name to her, the doctor could really listen and learn what kind of person she had been in earlier times and of her distress at becoming an almost anonymous resident in an unsavoury institution.

LAURA

She was referred to me by my partner who had been making no progress in treating her depression. I arranged to have a long interview with her to find out what it was all about and I've had two sessions together with her and her husband since then. They have a child now aged about one and they've been married for five years. She is a stockbroker and has worked half-time since the baby was born. She is very mixed up about being a businesswoman or a housewife and has been pretty miserable ever since the baby was born. Her husband has to travel a lot for his work, so is never there when she wants him. Well, she is a rather horsey person, in charge and managing everything. She is quite obsessional, but can't get around to actually doing any work, particularly when her husband is away. She seemed to be afraid of not being in control, but didn't seem to be all that depressed now that she had decided to put off having another baby.

Well, after the first session, I offered to see Laura together with her husband to try to focus on what was happening between them and perhaps also because I felt a bit put off by the way she seemed to be managing everything, including the way I had tried to work with her. He seemed to be terribly insensitive but quite concerned about her; a bit wet and out of his depth. But she was a real surprise. When we started talking about having a baby, she suddenly looked very feminine and almost attractive. It turned out that my invitation for them to come and see me had got them talking at home and they were now actually planning to have another baby.

The doctor felt discomfort at being 'managed' by his business-like patient and she created an impression of being in charge in a rather masculine way. Her husband was an insensitive, but affectionate man who was never there when he was needed. Yet when they came together to discuss their problems, the doctor suddenly saw Laura in a completely new way. She looked feminine and attractive and able to plan having a new baby. This was a new dimension of her personality, for the doctor had so far only seen her as a tough organized businesswoman who had achieved success in her male-dominated profession but was having depressed feelings after childbirth. She could now be seen as someone who was also very feminine, whose dilemma lay in her ambivalence about allowing herself to be feminine and frail as well as being businesslike and obsessionally efficient. The sudden observation of how different she looked gave an important insight into where her difficulties lay and pointed out what had to be talked about next, although she and her husband had already started talking at home about their plans. The doctor's new view put him in the picture and in closer touch with how things really were.

MARY

I've got two sisters in the practice. Jean has hypertension. She has two children and her husband has just had a vasectomy. I know her very well. Jean's sister, Mary, has a slight deformity of her spine and some time ago I referred her for physiotherapy and to see an orthopaedic surgeon, but I hardly know her at all. They both look rather similar and my secretary had given me the wrong cards. When Mary came limping in to see me, I said, 'Oh dear, you aren't Jean, are you?' and she said, 'No, I'm Mary, Mary Price, the one that lives alone.' Although she spoke quite casually, just enough to identify herself as the single one, I felt she was giving me an important message, in a way she wasn't quite aware of at the time.

The patient realized that to the doctor she was known as 'Jean's sister', a rather plain woman with a limp. Presumably others saw her that way too. Her complaints were of feeling tired and having backache, but the doctor might well have missed the underlying depression if he had failed to pick up the sad acceptance in the words 'I'm the one who lives alone.'

Most doctors encounter several patients every day who are ready to talk, but not always when they are ready to listen. This patient's almost unconscious remark highlighted the difference between her life and her sister's. This was exactly the area that was upsetting her and the wrong notes turned out to be a lucky accident which primed the doctor to her needs. It then turned out that she was as ready to talk about her personal life now as he was to listen.

JANE

I've been seeing her sporadically for some time because she is one partner of an unconsummated marriage. They're both in their early thirties and have been married for about ten years and have never had full intercourse in all that time. Jane had talked to me about it before. She had brought up the subject and she seemed to be the more enthusiastic of the two – I have seen her husband as well – but they have both said that their relationship was a good one. In fact, I see them round the place doing their shopping and talking in a way which suggests they get on well together. Anyway, I think I said at an earlier stage, 'why now? What made you get suddenly interested after all this time?' She said, 'well, I'm not all that bothered about whether we have sex or not, but I'd really like to have a baby.' They do cuddle and touch each other, but so far neither of them have been terribly interested in going further than that. I'd asked a bit about her own childhood and about her mother's pregnancy and she had told me that her mother had actually died in childbirth, giving birth to her younger sister. She had been brought up by aunts who had helped her father out. So having got that information, which was obviously important, I didn't really know what to do with it. There didn't seem any way at the time that I could use it helpfully. So I talked with them about the purely technical side of sexual intercourse and suggested that they read a book which I'd found helpful with other patients and I said, 'come back again next week.' But the sort of response I got was, 'well, a week is a bit too soon. We'll come back when we're ready, perhaps in a month or something like that.' So I would see them sporadically, usually when Jane felt it was time to come again. Usually the reason for coming again was for sleeping tablets. Each time she comes after a long interval, she begins by saying, 'I won't keep you long, I just want some more tablets.'

Well, she appeared again after a long interval and I gave her the sleeping tablets and then I thought I must do something about this marriage of theirs and this lack of sex and the baby she presumably still wants. Then I remembered the bit about her mother dying and I thought . . . I don't know why I decided to say something about that, but I did. I said, 'do you miss your mother a lot still?' She burst into tears and said that it was the anniversary of her mother's death and she'd actually just come from the cemetery where she'd been visiting her mother's grave. So it was quite a moment. In fact I said when she had dried her tears, it was interesting that after quite a long gap she'd come on this particular day, straight from her mother to see me.

The doctor knew this patient pretty well. He was familiar with her marriage and its problems and had been frustrated in his attempts to help. He had fallen into a pattern of giving her sleeping pills whenever she asked for them, although he really would have liked to help her to wake up into a fulfilled marriage. Then for the first time he felt driven to ask a completely focal question, outside the range of their usual talk about sexual performance and marital relationships. The bullseye was hit so accurately that the mood changed and tears were shed. The meaning of her unconsummated marriage and of her mother's death in childbirth was still unclear, but the weight of feelings for her lost mother and saddened childhood suddenly became present. For that moment, her doctor understood her and she knew that he had felt how sad she was and was able to help her put it into words. There were doubtless some clues of which he was unaware that led the doctor to make the remark that he did. There may also have been powerful impulses that pulled the patient to visit her doctor immediately after visiting her mother's grave. What mattered was that both were able to focus on feelings of lifelong importance for the patient. These may perhaps have been slowly seeking expression in the doctor–patient relationship for some time, but at that moment were close enough to the surface to be reached.

The traditional medical interview starts with a careful history of the complaint, followed by a systematic examination of the patient, leading to a diagnosis and the ordering of appropriate treatment. In our cases, each of the doctors was following the conventional technique, but then suddenly came off the professional pedestal and became aware of what was happening between himself and the patient. Learning about the patient's condition was replaced by experiencing what the patient was feeling. The doctor was suddenly engaged in the situation rather than studying it from outside.

What factors make a doctor change gear like this? Our cases share some common aspects even though they were treated by different doctors. In each example, there was dissonance within the consultation;

some unexpected reaction to suggest something was going on of which the doctor was unaware. Mrs Isaacs was seeking help from a doctor who was not yet on her side, indeed he didn't even know who she was. This doctor was able to appreciate the relevance of his own confusion to the old lady's situation and suddenly he was able to realize how lost she was feeling. Although in Laura's case, the doctor had allowed time for an initial long interview, he had been rather disconcerted by her brusque efficiency and professional competence. It was when she and her husband were talking about the possibility of having another baby that the doctor suddenly saw how she could be sexually attractive. Only then did he really understand the depth of her ambivalence; how to be an efficient and competitive businesswoman and a feminine wife and mother. When Mary consulted her doctor, he had the wrong notes, but despite being disconcerted by having to get the right ones, was alert to the overtones of her poignant statement that was aimed simply at identifying herself to him. Finally, Jane's doctor had expected to prescribe sleeping pills and perhaps struggle a bit more with the usual topic of sexual inadequacy. Suddenly he found himself catapulted into the immediacy of tears and almost lifelong unresolved grieving. He became more in touch with her true emotional world and gave up his stereotype of how he thought she ought to be feeling.

It seems that the doctor suddenly observes that what the patient is saying or how the patient is behaving no longer fits with what he expects. The doctor can either decide not to notice or deliberately try and look at this with more attention. Indeed the patient may have such pressing demands that the doctor feels unable to avoid the issue any longer. Sometimes something just happens and the doctor then has to stay with the situation and struggle to be aware of the overtones. Sensitive listening and being willing to react openly and spontaneously are the important skills. The ability to accept muddle is invaluable and doctors trying to work in this way have to learn not to try to sort out all the details, but to tolerate situations just as they are.

The daily dilemma is, of course, to distinguish which patients actually need to be heard in this way. After all, everybody has unresolved difficulties and not all of these need the doctor's ear. A doctor may feel that the patient's state is one that can be handled best by simply being a good technical physician without considering the wider aspects. Doctors differ greatly in their interests and aptitudes and every doctor, no matter how sensitive, is limited in his capacity to take on problems. Doctors cannot afford to be overwhelmed by an excessive burden of insoluble disasters any more than their patients. Yet patients are entitled to be treated appropriately. Family doctors have to consider their patients' circumstances as well as their diseases.

They need to develop sensitivity to the subtle nuances of patients' feelings so as to keep in touch with the whole of their patient's condition. Although this may take time, in the long run it must be an economical way of caring for people if it avoids excessive prescriptions for tranquillizers, unnecessary antibiotics, or unsuitable referral for specialist investigation. These are all very poor substitutes for proper understanding. The essence of our craft lies in achieving the right balance.

4
The touch on the tiller
Oliver Samuel and Cyril Gill

Most general practice consultations are quite brief. The kind of work that can be done in this setting depends critically on the context in which it takes place. General practitioners are readily available to help people in difficulties and, as there is very little stigma attached to 'going to the doctor', they are widely used. Although we live in a time of great social mobility and some doctors find that a large part of their practice population changes every year, most general practitioners stay in the same practice, looking after the same community, for the whole of their professional careers. Many patients still keep with the same doctor and together they face birth, growing up, marriage, illness, and eventually death. The very brief interviews that are usual in general practice have to be seen in this context. An unknown patient may seek help from a new doctor, or the consultation may be a brief but important episode in a life-long relationship. Both kinds of contact can help a patient, but the way the doctor copes with a patient he has known for a long time will be quite different from the way he approaches someone he hardly knows at all.

The following discussion looks beyond the detailed components within single consultations to the way important episodes fit into a relationship developed over long periods of time. The two cases described here concern patients whose doctors had known them for many years. In each case the doctor builds on his previous knowledge of the patients and their relationship to him but also attempts to stay open to new communications which will develop the picture further and deepen his accessibility to their needs.

ROSE
A 60-year-old lady attended the doctor with widespread patches of itchy erythema. She was all red and angry because the doctor had kept her waiting rather a long time. She brushed aside the doctor's apology. 'All I want is a letter to the hospital to sort out this rash.' The assumption that the doctor had no other part to play seemed

intentionally insulting. However, the doctor contained his own irritation. He remembered that she had been somewhat hostile before, but he had come through it successfully in the end. With a little persuasion she let him examine her. He asked if she had eaten anything unusual, worn any new clothes, or used new washing powders? She was very off-hand in her replies. What about bath salts? She scowled impatiently and the doctor felt very self-conscious. He was ill at ease and firing questions, while she was giving nothing away. He tried even harder. Had she been overworked or a little tired lately? She looked as though she was going to burst. He stopped trying altogether and said meekly that of course she could have a skin specialist if she wanted, but there would be a delay of about three weeks. She must have seen that he was trying, and perhaps he had been punished enough, because she suddenly melted and admitted there had been trouble lately. She described an office row, one of those triangular affairs between secretaries and employers which seem inevitable at times. He sensed her bitterness and hurt pride, and just nodded while she let out a gush of anger. He knew that she had few friends, and the office was an important part of her life. She had looked after a difficult and demanding mother too much and too long for her own good, and the doctor had shared this care too. Her mother had in earlier times done the same for her own mother. There was a legacy of frustration and bitterness which passed down the generations, but this patient had no family to lean on, no husband or children. Also she had no training to match her undoubted intelligence and potentialities. When her mother died she had shared all this with the doctor, but never let him refer to it again. The frustration and bitterness, which rightly or wrongly she attributes to her life with her mother, has left her vulnerable to insults, real or imagined, in her office or the doctor's waiting room. On a previous occasion she had attended with gastritis several times, and he had investigated and prescribed for her with no effect, until he discovered that her younger married sister was over here from Dublin. She had come because she wanted to visit London, but had never bothered to come when she would have been able to help. The patient was ashamed of voicing such petty thoughts to her sister or to anyone other than her doctor. She knew this medical relationship was confidential, but she still needed to make him feel rather useless before sharing her feelings. He had not seen her after that interview until the present one.

In the interview about the rash, it was clear to them both that resentment was again at the centre of the picture. It fitted her past, the rash, the row in the office, and the tension in the interview. The doctor showed her that he understood why the office row had been so painful. She agreed to try his prescription for the rash, though she probably did not need it. She did not mention the specialist again.

An interview in which the doctor and patient had remained on different wave-lengths would have failed. This interview was at the right depth. Resentment is not a very fundamental diagnosis, but it is adequate in the circumstances, and represents a level which the doctor and patient agree together. This lady chooses to live with her tensions, letting them out only when they are too intense. She does not want to face them and could not change herself very much. Feelings of failure and resentment lie in wait for her all the time. Her relationship to the doctor is one of mixed rivalry and dependence and she needs to humble him before she consults him, yet there is no-one else that she could possibly let know about her true feelings.

In the interview described, the doctor has helped her to look at her resentments. Has she just blown off steam, and returned to her previous level of tension? Does the doctor represent someone she needs in her life, from time to time? The doctor has found out a little more about her and has learnt to respond with more assurance. Has she too learnt a little about herself with a slight resolution of her internal tensions? It is hard to predict the outcome for this patient as other events, retirement perhaps, will soon intervene. The doctor could plan to get her to look at her ideas of self-fulfilment and re-evaluate them. Unfortunately, she is most unlikely to allow anyone to plan anything at all. She might come and use the doctor entirely differently next time. The patient holds most of the cards in this sort of work, though the doctor may get her to play a slightly different game with them.

SIMON AND GERALD

Simon is aged 67 and a portrait painter. He's been known to his doctor for years. He is homosexual and lives with Gerald who is three years older. Gerald is very unhappy because he is ageing and every birthday reminds him of the passage of time. By contrast Simon is bright and carries his age well. He is also rather more successful professionally than Gerald. They used to have a sexual relationship, but now although they remain very close, that has ceased some time ago. When Gerald last came in he was rather desperate and slightly grotesque. He is always excessively displaying and narcissistic. The doctor felt embarrassed by him and Gerald then said, 'it sounds so silly, I know you are going to laugh at me,' adding, 'my balls are shrinking,' and he burst into tears. The talk quickly turned to the business of ageing and how he hates it. He always steers away from looking at himself and said something about how young and marvellous the doctor was looking. But his pathos is clear in seductive statements of that sort.

Shortly after, Simon came to the surgery. He started by saying that everyone in the waiting room was coughing, but he was fine. He had come to talk about his mother who was in an old people's home and he wanted to have her moved to one in London so she could be visited more regularly. After discussing this he added, 'what are we going to do about Gerald? If it wasn't for Gerald I could travel, but he never wants to go anywhere. He wouldn't let me fly, you know. He would be so frightened in case something awful would happen to me.' Asked about ageing, the theme that dominates Gerald's consultations, Simon said, 'well I feel young and gay. I'm all right, but Gerald is really limiting me, although I do care for him a lot.' The doctor, suddenly feeling that this was important for him, said, 'perhaps you need that limit, perhaps he is not letting you fly off the handle.' Simon thought a bit and suddenly seemed to agree and said, 'maybe I'm feeling young because Gerald is older than me. Of course, I wouldn't do without him for the world.'

As the group talked about his case we found as soon as one or other of this extraordinary pair was mentioned, we immediately talked about how the other would react. We accepted them as a married couple of ageing homosexuals. As in *The Picture of Dorian Gray*, Gerald stayed at home and showed the ugly changes wreaked by passing time and suffered all the fears for both of them, while Simon maintained his vitality somewhat at the expense of his increasingly crabby stay-at-home partner.

The relationship that each had with the doctor seemed a vital prop for both. His understanding of their symbiosis enabled him to help them understand and cope with each other that bit more tolerantly. The episode reported here is of one occasion when the doctor showed Simon how he understood not only his feelings for Gerald, but also, despite the protestations of health, how he too needed to be restricted by Gerald's limited range of activities; how he was dependent on Gerald despite the outward appearance of being frustrated by him.

It is not difficult to understand how such a fragile couple benefit from the continuing tolerance and understanding of their doctor. This relationship has developed over many years and has been built up from many consultations such as those described. Being composed of short episodes of five to ten minutes in the course of busy surgery sessions, the cumulative development of knowledge and understanding of these patients has steadily progressed over a long time. As in the first case, the doctor's ability to respond accurately to the present situation is the direct outcome of spending time in understanding the patients a little bit better each time they come for help. This unique way of working is the essence of general practice and is quite unlike the relatively brief, though at times more intensive, case work of social workers or psychotherapists. In the second case it is important that the doctor is growing older along with his patients, for they have all known each other for years. Gerald's comments about how young the doctor looks is understood for the poignancy with which the observation is felt, both by the patient and his doctor, as are the pathetic seductive nuances. Each consultation can afford to be brief, for so much has been said before and is taken as understood. The work proceeds almost from where it last stopped, once the immediate business of the day has been dealt with.

How accurate was the doctor's comment about Simon's need for Gerald to limit his wish to travel and be 'young and gay'? Did it help either of them readjust to the realities of the passage of time that seemed such a source of distress? Fortunately, our group continued to hear reports about them both for over a year. At first they came often and manoeuvred the doctor into seeing them together. The material discussed with them separately was shared and acknowledged by both of them as right. Then Gerald developed alarming symptoms due to severe arthritis and became very agitated by the thought of becoming immobile. He needed a great deal of support and protection. Simon started coming more often with a whole series of minor problems; senile warts, backache, and the need to deny he was feeling older. He was much more relaxed about Gerald, however, attributing this to yoga. It was worth noticing that he still needed to tell the doctor about it too. He also seemed to want the doctor to join with him in telling Gerald to eat more sensibly. Gerald came one day and cried about the thought of his lifelong lack of professional success. He told, with much shame, of a fantasy of his own funeral when everyone realizes how much they really needed him.

The important moments of these consultations slightly changed the degree and quality of understanding between each of the patients and their doctor. This has steadily developed and matured over the years that they have known each other. The doctor responds to tears and denial, to seduction and rejection, and tries to understand the context in which it all happens. He allows Simon to see how much he depends on Gerald, then works with them together in a joint interview to help them digest this aspect of their ageing relationship, trying to help them move more honestly towards whatever may happen to them next. Their distress and refusal to accept growing old is one of the reasons behind Gerald's alarm when he develops symptoms of arthritis. This has to be taken into account while arranging the appropriate medical treatment. The doctor doesn't take over the management of the patients' lives. He acts with discretion and subtlety and, like a helmsman, touches the tiller and makes an important readjustment to the course and the trim of the sails so as to keep the momentum and line, but without showing much external evidence of what has happened. Simon still denies he is ageing, but somehow feels free to attend more often about minor ailments that might threaten his state of health. The doctor is better able to tolerate this as he knows more about the meaning of the complaints. Gerald develops arthritis and, as well as being given competent medical treatment, has to be comforted, mothered almost, to come to terms with this latest confirmation of his physical deterioration. The developing understanding that the doctor uses enables him to accomplish two tasks. It ensures that the patients feel the genuineness of his concern so that their feelings of isolation are shared by at least one other important person. It also enables the doctor to keep interested and involved in the mundane symptoms and temperamental storms of two very demanding and potentially tedious old men. Instead of getting fed up with them, they stand out for him as sad and fascinating people.

The kind of work described here is a long way removed from formal psychoanalytic psychotherapy from which it nevertheless derives. In both these cases, the patients present an inextricable mixture of physical complaints and psychological distress; illnesses and reactions reflecting each other in the most intimate way. It is only the family doctor to whom these patients can turn for this kind of care. Most of the interviews with the patients were brief yet, in both cases, the doctor's relationship with the patients had lasted for years. Each separate episode adds a further dimension to the depth of understanding the doctor is able to use in coping with both emotional crises and physical disease. This kind of work engages the doctor's concern and makes working with such patients worthwhile despite their apparently excessive demands for trivial and time-consuming attention.

5
Conflict or collaboration?
Marie Campkin and Erica Jones

It seems curious, in describing the transactions between doctor and patient, how much use we make of the language of the battlefield. The doctor and patient share a common interest in trying to improve the patient's health and ameliorate his symptoms, yet the process is commonly depicted in terms of conflict: defence, resistance, engagement, confrontation, and withdrawal.

'At that stage I was fighting back a bit . . . I don't think I made a frontal assault.'

'Is it a submission or a strategic withdrawal?'

'She was so challenging, it was difficult not to wrestle with her.'

'At the end of the interview the doctor was left feeling that both he and the patient had won a Pyrrhic victory.'

(excerpts from the group discussion)

To some extent this is because consultations in which progress is straightforward are unlikely to be reported in a working group like ours. The cases we were studying were those in which difficulties had been experienced but where some degree of change was occurring. Every doctor also has a personal catalogue of unreported 'chronic' cases, whose apparently static condition seems to constitute a burden to be borne by doctor and patient until parted by death. They are not necessarily patients with recognized chronic illnesses, though this may be part of the picture, but those with whom the doctor seems unable to make progress either in the resolution of their problems or in the development of his relationship with them. The resulting frustration of both parties may be endured with patient stoicism or fought with angry recriminations, or something between the two.

One encouraging aspect of the work is the way in which occasionally a patient like this unexpectedly moves and, at least for a while, there is a sense of change and a lightening of the burden. A greater understanding of the factors concerned may enable the doctor to do something about some of the other unprofitable relationships in which he is engaged, or perhaps he might discover how to prevent the 'difficult' case deteriorating into a 'chronic' one.

We should therefore ask what the relevant factors are in the doctor–patient relationship which determine whether it is to be a collaborative enterprise or a combat arena. It is tempting to look at the patient and formulate a series of reasons why he may be failing to co-operate – his personality, his defences, his aggression, and so on. Clearly, however, resistance may also be on the doctor's side and it is his professional task to become aware of his own defences and modify them so as to assist the patient to do the same, rather than to expect the patient to change without help.

MRS FRIEDMAN

The patient and her doctor have been sparring partners for years. She is over 80, an Austrian refugee who has suffered much. In the past she was a victim of Nazism and latterly she has had severe arthritis and depression. Her attendance, usually accompanied by her husband who seems to regard the doctor with some fellow feeling, heralds, 'a long and fairly painful conversation which ends with the patient prescribing her own treatment and the doctor feeling ground down by her grumbles'.

Some years ago she was anxious to have spa treatment in Germany for her arthritis. She understood this to be available under the National Health Service if a specialist recommended it and she felt the Germans owed it to her. The doctor was sceptical but agreed she should pursue her enquiries. Confronted then with the demand that he should sign the required documents, he took refuge quite truthfully in the fact that as he was not a specialist he was not eligible to do so. He agreed to refer her to a consultant, but did not go out of his way to choose one who was likely to comply, so perhaps was not altogether surprised when the plan fell through.

Subsequently, with her arthritis worsening, she reluctantly acqui-esced to his persuasion to have a hip replacement operation. As might have been predicted this proved to be 'not a disaster, but less than a success'. Four months after, the patient came to report that her pain was as bad as ever and to reproach the doctor yet again for his failure to have provided her with the treatment which in her view could have avoided the need for the unsatisfactory operation.

She went on to suggest that maybe she should go on a lecture tour, to tell British doctors about the benefits of continental spa treatment. The doctor was at a loss for words. She leaned forward and said, 'I am a horrible person, aren't I?' to which he replied, 'not entirely!' The patient grinned and left on the arm of her husband who was heard muttering, 'not entirely, not entirely, that's good.'

Several of the group recognized one particular aspect of this case, having experienced themselves the feeling of vicarious guilt which seems to complicate the relationship with survivors of persecution. They are often demanding and impossible to satisfy, while the doctor feels a special need to be a 'good' doctor to make up to them for past cruelties.

The group sympathized with the doctor's sufferings at the hands of this difficult patient, but they also felt for the patient in her resentment at being deprived of the treatment she trusted and being obliged instead to have surgery that didn't work. There was appreciation for the aptness and honesty of his response – 'not entirely' – at once acknowledging the patient's admission that she treats him badly but also his grudging regard for the saving grace of her sense of humour. (In the discussion he recalled a previous occasion when, having told him in a mood of depression that she was going to commit suicide, she had returned the next day and announced, 'The execution has been postponed.')

No doubt this combination of anger and sardonic humour has contributed to her survival through the vicissitudes of her life. She may be fortunate too to have a doctor who can also survive, bloody but unbowed beneath her assaults, even admitting to a sneaking fondness for her (and perhaps this describes her husband as well). Yet their antagonism can at times be destructive and unfortunate in its effects.

Had she been less dictatorial with her demands in general, he might have been better able to unbend a little in the matter of the spa treatment. Had he done this and it had proved helpful, he would have shared the credit. If it had failed, she could hardly have blamed him and in the event of her still needing the subsequent operation, the difference in her attitude might have made for a more favourable outcome.

Still it is understandable that the doctor feels a need to maintain his authority with this patient. It would not benefit her to have a doctor whom she can treat as a doormat, nor could he accept such a role in what must continue to be a long-term relationship. We wondered whether this interview with its brief moment of mutual appreciation would have any lasting effect. There seemed no likelihood that the patient would change, but the relationship might become a little more sympathetic or the doctor better able to tolerate her complaints in the light of this incident. The effect of having discussed the patient in the group may help the doctor to act on his improved understanding in his future dealing with her.

One positive aspect of the relationship between this patient and her doctor is the real mutual respect which underlies their apparent antipathy. A disturbing but persistent theme to emerge from our work was that a degree of contempt for the patient by the doctor can be a significant feature of their relationship, perhaps more often than we like to admit. When the point was first made by Enid Balint, it was received with dismay and some disbelief by the group, but the truth of the observation has important implications for our work.

'Can I tell you what I think changes? I think doctors stop being so contemptuous of patients. The first time round there's quite a bit of contempt in the doctor for the patient. When you bring a case to the group, the other doctors are not contemptuous and there's a kind of respect which comes in.'

The word 'contempt' has a somewhat pejorative ring, but if we consider Simone Weil's definition in *Waiting on God* (1951), 'Contempt is the contrary of attention,' we can see how our involvement and preoccupation with problems and traditional diagnostic labels can sometimes interfere with our paying due attention to the person in whom they occur.

'Whether you listen to them or not is something to do with respect or contempt. We sometimes start off by thinking we know exactly what they need – and we don't; and then we might change and actually listen to what they are saying and perhaps have some respect for that.'

For the origin of such an attitude one need look no further than to the traditional view of the doctor – specialist or general practitioner – as the wise, potent, authoritarian figure who knows best and whose mystique is part of his power. As Michael Balint pointed out, the method involving long interviews that had emerged from the earlier Balint groups perpetuated the role of the doctor as the leader or superior in the relationship. Referring to the doctor's conventional role, he wrote,

'These traditional functions assure the doctor of a safe feeling of superiority: it is he who knows more, to whom the patient turns with hope and trust, and who can prove by the success of his diagnostic skills that the trust in his superior knowledge and skills was justified.'   (Balint and Norrell 1973: 7)

The need to seek a change of focus becomes apparent with the failure of the illness-centred or doctor-centred approach to deal with problems arising in the patient's life and relationships, rather than in his systems and organs. Here the patient, not the doctor, is the 'one who knows more' and they must find a way of collaborating to explore the problem, while remaining within the context of the normal short consultation of everyday general practice.

The concept of patient-centred medicine is now widely accepted, but this has not eradicated the almost automatic initial assumption by the doctor of the superior role, with the patient occupying a position of relative insignificance. The hierarchical structure of the hospital system places the patient somewhere near the bottom of the pyramid – just above the medical and nursing students perhaps, but well below the porters and junior housemen. Yet even in the more egalitarian world of general practice the same assumptions are manifest in a more subtle form. That this also accords with the patient's view is illustrated by the apologetic attitude with which even seriously ill patients often approach their general practitioners – 'I don't like to take up your time, doctor', 'I know how busy you are', 'I'm sorry to be a nuisance' or on visits, 'sorry to drag you out'.

Before closer communication can take place, the doctor's mantle of superiority must be shed, making way for a more personal concern and respect. Initially, the doctor and patient meet as strangers, each measuring the other against expectations based on past experience. But most general practitioners know hundreds of patients at a time, and thousands over a period of years, whereas most patients only experience a few doctors in their lifetime. So it is not surprising if the doctor tends to categorize the patient – fitting him or her into a convenient mental compartment. The patient meanwhile is likely to be making a more simple judgement – is this doctor better or worse than my last one?

Sometimes it takes a long time and many meetings for the doctor to see the patient for the first time as a real person, in a moment of identification which may provide the key to the development of their working relationship. Since this usually takes place as part of the normal 'natural history' of the development of the doctor–patient relationship, it is worth trying to understand those situations in which its occurrence is unreasonably delayed. It was often the fact of a change in the doctor's perception from a stereotyped to a personal view of the patient that made the case an appropriate one to present – that is, one in which something new seemed to have happened.

HILDA

Hilda is a stout, matronly widow in her 70s who lives with her 50-year-

old, grossly obese, and mentally-handicapped daughter. The doctor
has known her for years and is aware that her husband, an army
officer, died abroad many years before. She has various long-standing
complaints about backache and abdominal pain and sees the doctor
occasionally for blood pressure checks and to have a bit of a grumble.
In between she has repeat prescriptions. The relationship with the
doctor could be described as cordial but superficial, and the traditional
diagnosis would be diverticular disease, moderate hypertension, and
arthritis.

On this particular occasion the doctor's attention was caught by the
patient's heavy-footed entry into the consulting room – somehow not
quite like her usual self. Her initial somatic complaints gave way to an
admission of feeling 'down'. Her daughter was in a prolonged sulk,
refusing to speak to her, and Hilda, mourning the first anniversary of
her brother's death, felt she might be 'losing her will to live.'

Trying to assess the extent of her depression, the doctor asked, 'do
you mean that when you go to bed, you wouldn't mind if you didn't
wake up again?' The patient replied, 'yes, of course.' The doctor said,
'have you ever felt you might harm yourself?' and she answered, 'no, of
course not.'

With a little encouragement, she went on to tell the doctor in vivid
detail about her husband's tragic death and her daughter's subsequent
breakdown, from which she had never recovered. After this she
reverted to describing her present problems – her flat, her 'Home
Helpless' who kept failing to turn up, and her abdominal pain. The
doctor examined her, advised about diet, and prescribed an anti-
spasmodic. The patient commented, 'it's nice to have someone to talk
to – you can't talk to the milkman,' and on reaching the door added, 'I
really feel much better.'

The doctor had been particularly struck by the disparity between her
ready admission of a wish to be dead and her categorical denial of the
possibility of acting on such a wish. This suggested a fresh view of the
patient as an upright woman with a strong sense of duty who would
continue to bear whatever burdens fate had in store for her.

She had admitted her need to talk to someone – 'not the milkman'
– but her daughter was not speaking to her and her brother was no
longer available. Having unburdened herself of some painful memories
she resumed her normal composure and departed, rewarding the
doctor for having listened with a complimentary parting remark. The
doctor was now feeling some real sympathy and indeed admiration for
her courage, and in summarizing the case for the group, formulated
the new working diagnosis in these terms: 'A dutiful mother, isolated

from her social and intellectual equals and bereft of her brother's support. Her daughter is like a "cuckoo in the nest" needing constant feeding but returning little reward.'

Certainly in the course of this interview Hilda herself has become a 'real person' to the doctor, but in the discussion it was clear that the daughter remains a nonentity. The 'cuckoo in the nest' simile was apt but a considerable degree of 'contempt' is implicit in it. The doctor's afterthoughts included, 'I was rather horrified to realize how I had dismissed the daughter as an enormous unattractive being whose infrequent attendances are mercifully brief, and how little I really know about her.'

A month or so later the patient returned with more physical symptoms but this time she seemed anxious in case there might be something seriously wrong. She mentioned that she was now the last of her family – 'her turn next, but not yet'. When the doctor referred to her daughter's health – no doubt out of guilt for previous omissions – Hilda mentioned the provisions she had made for her daughter's future care after her death.

A group member commented, 'I find myself thinking what a struggle it is for patients to get their doctors to find them interesting – but having managed it, it's provided an impetus which has carried on and you're willing to look at what's going on between her and her daughter in much more detail than before.'

'Perhaps that's the long-term effect of the "important moment" – the patient does "make himself interesting" and then any subsequent consultation has that extra spark.'

'What does that mean though – to be interesting to someone? Does it mean to be seen to be alive, to be a human being?'

There was one further interview reported another month later. On this occasion the doctor made an effort to avoid keeping the patient waiting, and the patient came in with a smile. After preliminaries about tablets and blood pressure, Hilda said she was going on holiday to her older, married daughter leaving her other daughter behind. She said, 'It's a real holiday – I don't have to do anything. But every time I go I think it will be the last time.'

The doctor looked up sharply. She said, 'Oh no, I don't mean that – it's just the travelling that's difficult – changing trains and no porters and so on.'

It now seems that the patient has progressed from 'losing her will to live', through anxiety about possible serious illness and death, to reassuring her doctor that she is not now worrying about her own death. In clinical terms this could be seen as a straightforward recovery from a period of depression following a bereavement. In human terms there is more to it, though the changes that have taken place seem modest enough: the doctor is more welcoming and more concerned, and the patient shows awareness and consideration for the doctor's feelings. She is no longer a 'repeat prescription' patient.

Both these cases involved elderly patients whose basic problems were unlikely to change a great deal. There is a possibility of improved understanding leading to some mellowing of the relations between doctor and patient. But there are often occasions when both the relationship and the problems are at a much earlier and less stable stage. Then the outcome of a particular consultation, or series of consultations, may have far-reaching effects and the doctor's ability to prevent his own or the patient's defences from interfering with the progress of the work may be crucial.

Interference with the work may take many forms. External circumstances such as pressure of time and interruptions, superficial distractions due to appearance or mannerisms, conscious reluctance to get too deeply involved, or unconscious resistance to the examination of certain aspects of the problem can all conspire to sidetrack patient and doctor into irrelevant diversions or unprofitable interactions. It may be by no means clear to the doctor which are the more profitable aspects of a transaction in which he is himself closely engaged at the time. This is where the opportunity of bringing the case for discussion in a group often helps to illuminate what is going on.

It is sometimes suggested that in attempting to penetrate the patient's defences the doctor may be exceeding his medical prerogative and making an unwarranted intrusion into the patient's privacy. It is true that a clumsy attempt to interrogate the patient about sensitive issues is unlikely to be productive and will provoke resentment. But if it is accepted that much of the illness presented to the general practitioner is of emotional or psychological origin it would be unrealistic to prohibit efforts to understand it on the grounds of possible trespass into a forbidden area.

However, just as one would not undertake an intimate physical examination without clinical justification, appropriate explanation, and the patient's consent, so the same principles must be applied in approaching the exploration of intimate areas of the patient's personal life. Like the physical examination it must be conducted with consideration and expertise so as to avoid causing the patient damage or undue distress. This is best achieved by trying to keep in tune with the patient's feelings and being sensitive to the nuances of his responses as the interview proceeds.

LESLEY

The encounter began inauspiciously, with the patient being fitted in as an 'extra' because the partner she was booked to see was unable to sign her passport application. The doctor, already well behindhand in a busy surgery, agreed to complete the form, but felt irritated when the patient, a 38-year-old woman whom she knew slightly, also started to complain about pains in her back. The doctor suggested that she should make a further appointment for this, to which the patient readily agreed.

Two days later she reappeared, unfortunately again at a time when the doctor was badly behind the clock. The presenting symptoms of long-standing neck and back pain and tiredness offered some temptation to keep things at the strictly physical level, but the doctor's dutiful enquiry about depression produced an unmistakable response. She felt bound to go further and invite the patient to talk a little about herself.

She was willing to talk about her work as a theatrical designer, but seemed reluctant to discuss her personal life. The doctor felt she was being fended off from the crux of the problem, but persisted and it gradually emerged that Lesley had undergone tubal surgery three years before, after years of infertility, only for her husband to have now lost interest in sex. She was at pains to assure the doctor that this didn't really matter, as there was some possibility that they might adopt a child. In any case, she understood that refraining from sex reduced the likelihood of getting cancer of the womb and she thought she might be at risk because she had had a cervical erosion.

At this point the doctor found herself embarking on a didactic explanation of why this idea was a misconception, at the same time becoming uncomfortably aware of its complete irrelevance to the patient's real needs. Cutting the lecture short, she pressed the patient to concede that there might be a connection between her total denial of distress about what must be a very painful area of her life – her childlessness and marital problem – and her overt symptoms of weariness and pain. Lesley admitted that she was unable to talk to her husband about it for fear of hurting him and though she had some friends she could 'have a grumble with', she could not tell them about this part of her life.

The doctor suggested she should come another day for a physical examination and to talk about the problem again.

In reporting the case to the group the doctor gave the traditional diagnosis as 'cervical spondylosis and depression' and the overall diagnosis as 'a sad woman who is denying her distress about her childlessness to protect her husband, but paying the price with physical and emotional symptoms.'

In discussion, the group puzzled about the apparent coincidence of her successful fertility treatment and the onset of her husband's loss of libido. Did he only want sex when he couldn't have children? We also wondered whether the doctor had been seduced by the patient's teasing – leading on and warning off – or was it she who had forced an entry through the patient's defences? If so, was it for the patient's benefit, or to satisfy the doctor's curiosity? 'A form for a passport to go travelling somewhere is an interesting start – but how much of the tour is what she wants to do and how much is what the doctor wants to hear?' It was suggested that the doctor may have signed not only a passport form, but adoption papers as well.

Inevitably the doctor approached the next interview a few days later with a private agenda of unanswered questions. The patient began by announcing that she had felt much worse after seeing the doctor. She had spent some time in thinking about her situation and had concluded that she had indeed had much to be unhappy about, including several matters not previously mentioned concerning her work and relationships with her family. As a result she had reached decisions about certain actions to relieve some of the pressures on herself and her husband.

The doctor was anxious to clarify the question of adoption and felt relieved that this seemed a distant prospect. The patient said her husband was even more anxious than she was that they should have a child, yet their fertility investigations had been allowed to drag on for years, apparently through lack of assertiveness on both their parts.

The promised physical examination proved, as expected, negative and some different tablets were prescribed for the back pain.

A few weeks later she returned, saying things were looking up. Her husband had made love to her and the pills were marvellous and had got rid of the pain. The doctor, who had felt initially that the patient might need long-term psychotherapy, was astonished at the speed with which she had begun to come to terms with her problems. It appeared that once she had accepted the idea of an emotional basis for her pain she was prepared to admit her unhappiness and fight it rather than be depressed. But there was a worrying feeling that maybe this was a little bit too good to be true.

The group commented that her relationship with her husband seemed rather like an older sister, protecting him and fighting his battles. Perhaps she felt the doctor had taken a similar protective role with her, allowing her for once to admit her own weakness and dependence. The doubt remained as to whether the result was a success or whether she had made a 'flight into health' to evade further scrutiny.

Some months later she attended for some minor complaint and reported that things had improved a good deal all round. She had only occasional pain, her work was going well, and the physical relationship with her husband had improved. Once she had become more open and assertive and less worried about hurting him, he in turn had become more responsive.

Then, almost exactly a year after the initial interview, the doctor was puzzled to see on the appointment list the patient's surname with a strange Christian name. Expecting this to be some visiting relative, she was confounded by the entry of husband and wife with a very new baby, just acquired for adoption. They were obviously delighted and the doctor's main hesitation in sharing their pleasure was anxiety lest any hitch might occur in the adoption procedure and apprehension for the enormous disappointment this would cause. However, the couple were extremely optimistic and the doctor could only keep quiet, with fingers crossed.

This scenario which started with a passport could be seen as a journey crossing a series of defensive frontiers. It begins with the doctor tempted by the constraint of time to postpone or avoid setting out at all, but impelled by conscience to proceed, the patient following but doubtful whether they are going in the right direction. The doctor is almost drawn into a cul-de-sac, but backtracks to get on the right road. The patient then agrees to the suggested route, proceeds a considerable distance on her own, and eventually manages to get her husband to come along with her. Suddenly they are joined by another traveller – the baby. Who knows where the road will lead now? It is the doctor who is cautious and would like to slow down, but she has now been left behind.

The nature of the defences and resistances of doctors and patients was a periodic theme for our consideration.

'It's a defensiveness, isn't it? It can show in all sorts of ways – keep off, or be excessively nice so that you don't have to face whatever awful feelings you have.'

'The change brought about by training is surely a shedding of resistance, dropping a few barriers to extend one's repertoire, becoming more available to a wider range of people.'

There are a number of mechanisms whereby patient and doctor can keep each other at arm's length. The concept of 'distance' is important, since the relationship is a dynamic affair in which the movement of either party alters the space between them. One could postulate that there is an optimum 'distance' for a particular patient and doctor, at which point the tasks of communication, diagnosis, and treatment are best facilitated. This point is at a fragile equilibrium which can easily be disturbed by further movement on either side, so that profitable consultations may be followed by an unproductive period, just as a seemingly impenetrably bogged-down relationship can move into a more favourable phase.

If the distance is too great, the patient remains stereotyped – fat girl, deaf old lady, alcoholic, neurotic, and so on. If it is too close, the doctor's involvement with the patient as an individual may interfere with the need to maintain a critical professional detachment.

Some of the permutations of defence and distance could be summarized under the headings: fight, fright, and flight. Where there is mutual antipathy between doctor and patient in an atmosphere of 'fight', any movement tends to be of one against the other. The result will fall somewhere along a scale from confrontation, through armed neutrality and passive non-compliance to a simple agreement to differ. This makes for a disagreeable relationship in which 'important moments' are hard to come by as neither party wants to give way – rather as in the case of Mrs Friedman, reported above.

In a situation characterized by 'fright', there may be apprehension of the consequences of too honest a relationship and an implicit conspiracy to avoid painful areas. Superficially things may be pleasant and gratifying to patient and doctor as they move along side by side, maintaining the status quo. For progress to occur, the relationship may need to become less comfortable, less collusive, and more challenging, though this may prove too threatening to continue for long. The report about Lesley shows some of these features.

In the case of Hilda (and also Sarah in Chapter 8), it was the doctor's feelings of incongruity, surfacing during an apparently 'routine' consultation, which resulted in a more intense and intimate exchange for a time as the doctor struggled towards a better understanding. Afterwards the relationship reverts to a more mundane level which is easier to tolerate, but it will never be quite the same as before, for something useful has been achieved.

A third variation is when patient and doctor are moving away from each other in 'flight' – the doctor perhaps in despair at the insolubility of the problems and the failure of previous efforts to get closer – the patient in disgust at the doctor's inability to change anything. Both may retreat behind the barricades, until such time as some external event occurs to alter the situation for them, or one of them terminates the relationship.

MARTHA
The doctor's picture of her was of a 'sad, shrivelled lady', divorced years ago from a violent husband and left alone to bring up two severely mentally handicapped teenagers after her three older children had left home. The doctor had cared for the family for years, dealing with Martha's headaches and menstrual problems, providing a sedative for the daughter's tantrums, and hearing about the son's frightening and uncontrollable rages. Martha always looked unhappy, spoke in an unemotional monotonous voice, had a rather grey colour – and the doctor 'felt impotent to penetrate the thick wall of patiently borne misery, expressed, if at all, with the words "it's very difficult, doctor." '

Then one day she came to the doctor and said 'I'm feeling so ill, so awful!' But she actually looked a little better, more animated, with a little colour in her grey face. With encouragement she began to talk about the death of her ex-husband a few weeks before, after two years' illness, speechless and choking to death with a growth in his gullet. She recalled her difficult life with him, his violence getting worse with each child, and the handicapped son seeming the last straw. On one occasion she had locked herself in her bedroom, and when he began to break down the door, she had jumped from the second-floor window to escape, injuring her spine and ankle, which had never been right since. Soon afterwards they were divorced. The older children felt bitter about him, but she said wistfully that they had had some happy times before the children came, and though she had been frightened of him for so many years she had felt sorry for him in his illness and had sent her daughter to visit him.

The doctor was amazed at all this information after years of monosyllabic non-communication. Martha returned by invitation two days later and talked more frankly of her early life: how her husband had sexually assaulted the oldest daughter, who had then had a nervous breakdown; how the handicapped son had been fostered and had never forgiven her, and she had accepted his difficulties as a punishment; how she had later discovered her husband had also sexually assaulted the two youngest children. She began to weep, apologetically at first, but more freely with the doctor's acceptance.

In discussing the case, the group felt that somehow her husband's death had freed Martha from her inarticulate misery to allow her to express her sadness and to mourn all her losses – her failed marriage, her children's troubles, and her husband's painful death – at last. Perhaps the doctor's tolerance of her mute misery for five years had helped to make this present revelation of her feelings possible, and she might now begin to make a new life for herself.

She did not return for some time but her liberation, if that is what it was, seems to have had a powerful effect on the younger children. Some months later her son married a girl he had met at the Reading Centre. She too had problems, and could read less well than he did, but he spoke proudly of 'my wife' and seemed to be becoming more adult and responsible. The daughter had left school and achieved some independence with a simple part-time job, dressing more like a young woman rather than a little girl, and talking to the doctor 'without muttering into her lap'. Martha no longer fears her son – if he still has rages they are not directed at her – but she is frightened when she is alone in her flat, lest someone should break in.

Perhaps the most encouraging aspect of this last case is the fact that the years of apparently fruitless effort by the doctor to make contact with Martha's feelings have not been wasted. Somehow the foundations had been laid for the relationship to develop once the barriers finally fell, even though the doctor herself could do nothing more to bring this about. Without the groundwork, Martha might have had no-one to turn to when the flood of released emotion threatened to overwhelm her. Having tolerated the long period of frustration, the doctor was now able to provide the lifeline.

Without similar efforts by the doctor, in all these diverse situations, to recognize the nature of the defensive stalemate and take appropriate action, too often a difficult relationship will deteriorate into an uneasy mixture of collusion and contempt. Can it be that these two hazards are two sides of the same coin? It is a curious fact that sometimes the most contemptuous thing a doctor can do to an aggressive or demanding patient is to give him exactly what he has asked for – referral, investigation, or drug – knowing that it is not what he really needs, with a mental note that it serves him right. But we may be behaving similarly, albeit with different sentiments, when we collude with more congenial patients in order to be 'nice', to show a good bedside manner, to keep their approval by letting them have their own way rather than challenging them about what they ask for.

By learning about the pattern of these defensive interactions and becoming more aware of them, the doctor can improve his ability to identify and deal with them when they occur in practice. This may mean either taking the initiative and relinquishing his own defences a little, to encourage the patient to follow his example; or confronting him with his own view of the situation; or sometimes tolerating frustration without despair until something turns up to bring about a change.

6
Moments of change
Andrew Elder

A general practitioner who sits behind his desk resolutely hoping to make all his patients better will soon be exhausted or disillusioned. The doctor in general practice has to learn to live with his patients in a much more unchanging world than often both would wish. The doctor is frequently in the dark, getting glimpses of his patients from time to time, being careful not to find out too much, being content to find the right distance for the patient and himself; sometimes taking the initiative and at other times needing to be more restrained. The frustrations of this work have to be borne, just as uncertainty and hopelessness also have to be, in order to allow other possible changes to occur.

The purpose of this chapter is to study to what extent these two worlds – the doctor's and the patient's – meet in moments of understanding between the two. How much of a real communication can there be? How much of the patient's world can the doctor appreciate? And if for a moment there is a contact, how does it affect the relationship afterwards? What changes and in whom? These are difficult questions to study in any setting. In general practice they are doubly so because of the varied and transitory nature of the contacts.

There may be many moments in consultations when the doctor more or less successfully hears what the patient is communicating and tunes in. But occasionally more significant interviews occur, which contain a moment when the doctor's whole view of the patient may alter; a pivotal point around which a change in their relationship occurs.

One of the doctors reported a contact with a patient who in many senses might be thought a 'hopeless case'. She had seen him just two or three days previously and the interview turned out to last about twenty minutes.

RALPH
He's aged 63. He's been with the practice for about four years and I

know him to be a long-standing alcoholic who pops in and out of the liver unit at the local hospital. He's one of a number of patients who one feels is probably somewhat unhelpable. He had had a recent brief admission with a bleeding gastric ulcer. He came in and said he'd got a cough but wasn't in any way incapacitated, but obviously he had had a drink sometime that day and so really I was quite prepared to treat his cough and not do anything very much else, but I decided that perhaps one should once again talk about this drinking. He said that in 1978 there'd been some kind of group formed at the hospital which he had attended regularly for more than two years and with that support he'd managed to keep off the booze, but since then he couldn't do without his bottle of Martini because the withdrawal symptoms he'd got were so bad. He said he just feels as if he's strangled and can't breathe; knows that his days are numbered. I think he desperately wants to stop but is terribly frightened of this every-night feeling that he is choking. At some point I was beginning to feel more sympathetic to him and he was sort of warming up a bit and being more communicative, and said he was a homosexual and a psychologist had given him the name of a homosexual group in London . . . nothing to do with alcoholics, just as a kind of support group that he might get in touch with. I asked him if he'd ever tried Alcoholics Anonymous and he said he didn't care for it very much. He seemed really quite serious again about stopping drinking and I asked whether he would be willing to go into hospital again to be dried out. But he said that he couldn't possibly go into hospital at the moment because he was about to lose his present job. He's a storeman and has worked in a family firm for many years, but the firm is packing up and he has in fact got a new job to go to, starting on Monday. He said at sixty-three he obviously isn't going to get another offer and so he's very anxious to get to the job. As he gets bad withdrawal symptoms I thought I could tide him over a few days with Heminevrin (chlormethiazole), which isn't a drug I'm very familiar with or very happy about using. I knew he hadn't any family and I asked him if he had any homosexual friends or contacts and he said no he hadn't and it was a bit hard. He was very lonely, obviously. I sort of arranged that he would ring me up on Monday to tell me how he was and so on. As he was about to leave he reminded me gently that we'd forgotten about his cough which I was going to prescribe for. So I added an antibiotic for his chest. As he was going he said something about, 'I seem to have taken up a lot of your time.' It was actually twenty minutes. And he went off, looking quite cheerful and I felt quite cheerful about it at the end of the consultation. I felt a bit hopeful about him. But I don't know, I had after-thoughts.

This seems at first sight a fairly straightforward business. The doctor sees a patient and decides to perform what is asked of her and not enquire much further. Her first impression is that this man is something of a hopeless case. Her diagnosis might have been 'chest infection in a chronic alcoholic with poor prognosis'. However, as the doctor mentions later in the discussion, she had 'recently been successful with another patient with a long history of drinking' so perhaps this, together with the feeling of warmth she notices in herself, are sufficient to prompt her into making a few enquiries and listening a bit as the patient explains how important it is for him to hold on to his new job. A feeling of sympathy is aroused and the doctor's conscience stirred. 'Something he said to me, you know, I just felt that I couldn't deliberately shut my eyes to his enormous problem and just deal with his little problem.'

There is no dramatic change in the relationship here. The doctor's world and the patient's world do not seem particularly close, but there is a definite movement during the interview away from the original conception of a 'lonely homosexual alcoholic with liver failure' towards a person for whom the doctor arranges 'that he would ring me up on Monday to tell me how he was'. It is likely that the patient has had a lifelong experience of being rejected. He is not someone who would come expecting the doctor's individual attention and may well be rather ashamed or overwhelmed to receive it. One of the other doctors commented in the discussion, 'This is a man who gets pushed off, isn't it?' It is easy to imagine a busy doctor choosing to deal with such a case quickly in order to catch up on the morning surgery. However, this doctor has not been shocked by this man, nor fired with too great a zeal for reforming him. She has treated him as a person in need of help and not as just another alcoholic, accepting him in much the same way as many experienced general practitioners would have done.

As discussion of the case developed there seemed to be general agreement that what the doctor had achieved with this patient was valuable: 'this is getting the atmosphere right so that you can engage with the patient in a working sort of way.' Regardless of the fact that he may feel, 'Oh my God, she's talking about the booze I had!'

At the same time there was a persistent doubt that ran through the discussion. Could there have been another area of more intense contact between these two that never quite occurred? This other theme was opened by one doctor who remarked, 'I think that if you concentrate on trying to stop him drinking, you'll miss doing the really important work, the possible work, and I feel very gloomy about it.'

This possible work that came close to the surface but did not quite break into the open, seemed to be associated with the patient's terror of the night, his feeling of suffocation. This was the direction in which strong and immediate feelings seemed to lie. 'I think he needs to share just how absolutely intolerable it is looking at the night. He can cope with the day when he is working. It's just that he obviously dare not go to sleep without his bottle.'

The patient, lonely and frightened, is nearing death. He has probably been frightened of darkness, the night-time, and being alone, all his life. Could such a feeling be shared? What would have to happen in the doctor's mind to make such a sharing possible? Intellectual recognition that this was a likely aspect of the patient's experience would not be sufficient.

We often referred in our discussions to 'changing gear' and 'levels of engagement'. Perhaps we can see three or four possible 'gears' or 'levels' in this case.

A doctor could assess the situation pretty quickly and decide to give the minimum that is asked. He knows he has made that choice and does not feel too badly about it. He recognizes that he cannot do everything for everybody and keeps his head down when the outlook doesn't look too promising. The doctor reporting the case had probably adopted this approach on the first few occasions of seeing this patient.

Another level might involve a doctor seizing on the patient, regarding the chest infection as the patient's 'ticket of entry', and his alcoholism or possibly even his homosexuality as the 'real problem', as something general practitioners should be on the look-out for and 'manage'. He would take various 'appropriate' steps – withdrawal from alcohol first, then social support, homosexual counselling, etc; textbook management without much regard for the person. This doctor would be a little like a parent, who, facing the patient frightened at night, clutching on to his bottle, reacts by trying to take it away, saying 'That'll do you no good. You had better give it up.'

A more sophisticated approach might lead the doctor to see the patient as an unhappy man, feel some sympathy for his condition, and allow him time and human breathing space. This response is to the person, not the problem, and paves the way for making himself a useful doctor for the patient in the future. The parental voice this time is saying, 'I can see you're in a mess and do need your alcohol. I can accept that, and realize that it'd be more or less impossible for you to live any other way. It'd be nice if you could, but I'll be here if you can't. I'll encourage you if you do well and won't be too accusing or rejecting if you fail.' This seems close to the doctor's actual management.

A further possibility of a more intense contact, was the one mentioned earlier. This time the doctor goes along with the patient as

above, but also allows just enough of the patient's main communication, perhaps terror, into his own experience at that moment, to feel
something of his own terror of death and being left alone. Such an
experience may alter for some time the relationship between the doctor
and patient; with the doctor seeing the patient more vividly and
responding to him from a richer perspective, while the patient perhaps
also experiences the doctor in a different light.

Paradoxically such moments seem more likely to occur when
thoughts of change or 'changing things for the better' are furthest from
the doctor's mind.

In this particular case, it is clear from the follow-up reports that the
doctor did become someone that this lonely and unhappy man could
turn to for help. He did get into trouble with the new job and began
drinking heavily, but came to the doctor earlier than he might have
done and was admitted for 'drying out'. There was more and more
emphasis on his 'drinking problem'. He came often and had been seen
twenty-seven times in a year at the last follow-up report. The
relationship seemed to be settling into the kind doctor and the
unfortunate man. In one follow-up report there is mention of the
patient's dread of being found in a coma, taken for dead, and buried
alive.

None of the doctors who were in the group are trained psychotherapists and few have had experience of personal therapy or analysis. We
were, however, all experienced in the use of such psychotherapeutic
skills as are commonly used in general practice. We were not
concerned with describing the effects of these skills themselves. They
are part of the mature doctor's technical equipment, along with his
stethoscope, ophthalmoscope, or pharmacopoeia. We were more
interested in studying the tuning of a doctor's whole response to the
patient. In most cases the doctor had tried all his usual 'tricks'. These
were doomed because they lay within the restrictions of the present
relationship between the doctor and patient. If there was to be a
change it would be to bring the two into a greater area of contact with
each other, as seemed to occur in the following case.

STUART

The doctor had known Stuart, a young man in his twenties, for about
four years before discussing the case in the group and had usually
found him a rather exasperating patient. He described his previous
relationship with him in the following way: 'Irritating and unexpressive
– he looks incredulous and superior. I usually felt like shaking him but
instead had treated him with exaggerated caution – "kid gloves".' He

reported two interviews, almost a month apart, in which the usual pattern of their relationship seemed to change.

'He is a tall, rather expressionless, very superior sort of thin chap . . . who was a student when I first came across him a few years ago, when he was due to take some exams. He presented a lot of escalating anxiety before his exams and pulled out of them. I think this happened at least two or three times; very similar patterns, he came with insomnia and restlessness and lots of symptoms linked with anxiety which was focused entirely on his forthcoming exams.'

The doctor never felt effective at helping him with this and used to see him increasingly frequently as his exams approached, and ended up prescribing different and stronger tranquillizers, until Stuart would withdraw, go home, and things would calm down a bit until the following year. After this cycle recurred two or three times, the doctor himself felt desperate and referred the patient to a counsellor who worked in his surgery. She saw him weekly for a year and we used to discuss him from time to time. Exactly the same cycle returned. He left college and never got a degree. He took a temporary job as a driver at a local firm and is still there, two years later.

The doctor had later seen him when he had been found to have iritis and his firm wouldn't employ him until it was fully investigated and treated. He had become a frequent attender and continued to present his anxiety state in a way that made the doctor feel helpless. It was against this background of frequent consultations and with the doctor feeling stuck that he began his report of the more recent interviews.

He started with various physical symptoms, as though he'd never seen me before. Incredibly boring and very detailed and distant. He was very controlled but aggressive about doctors and things, telling a long story, with many minute physical symptoms: he had tingling sensations and had gone to the occupational health service who had said it was anxiety, and then he had gone to casualty and they'd given him some tranquillizers which he chucked across my desk in a very disparaging way. Then he'd gone home, and really he knows me well, up to his parents and seen their doctor who had given him a different tranquillizer and again the same sort of inadequate transaction was described.

The doctor clearly thinks that the patient should not be as dismissive of his efforts as this and should have responded more positively to his therapeutic endeavours, but the patient feels differently. He feels helpless and unhelped – and this feeling he successfully passes on to the doctor who now describes his mounting irritation.

I felt really furious with him and actually gave him a good sort of bashing, though in rather a covert way. I mean, I said how difficult he found it to trust anyone and how awful it must feel to him to have such useless doctors who couldn't help him and it must leave him feeling very helpless. He looked rather stunned and said he wasn't worried about anything. He had no worries. I then said that perhaps it wouldn't be a bad thing if he did, it wouldn't be such a disaster, instead of floating above it all the time. And he looked pretty stunned about that and I felt fairly bad after it and followed up saying, 'we must take your symptoms seriously,' and went through a careful physical examination. It was a full half-hour.

There was a gap of a month before the patient consulted the doctor again. He started by telling the doctor of his recent symptoms. The doctor commented that it was like exam-time again, but this time there were no exams. The patient responded by saying he was a bit worried about work and still being there, and had had a bit of trouble with his landlady. He liked the firm, finding the work enjoyable: 'The people are fun – though my parents are worried, they say, "ah, well, if you like it." '

I asked him whether his parents were always understanding with him, tolerant. He looked at me rather surprised and said, 'Yes, well, of course' . . . but looked down and talked for a bit and then said, 'yes, maybe what I do need is a bit of a kick up the backside.'

This provided a link back to the last interview and quite a sudden clue to the relationship. The doctor then said that he had felt that he had given him a bit of one last time, and that maybe he could survive a good kick now and then. The doctor was conscious of his own previously cautious and inhibited handling of the patient. He remarked to the patient that he had often felt rather intimidated by him and perhaps the patient had more power over things then he realized. This produced a definite reaction in the patient, quite unlike anything he had shown of himself before. This idea that he had been intimidating or that he was powerful shook him absolutely and then he sort of laughed and it was the first time I had seen this man really show some feeling. And he couldn't get over it. 'What?! Me?! Powerful?!' It just left him obviously with some sort of new idea about himself, and that was that interview.

What seems to have happened here? All the doctor's endeavours to change, reform, or cure the patient, whether by prescription, referral, or trying to understand his background have come to nothing. The patient remains firmly aloof. He brings along his mounting anxiety through symptoms and, as though detached from them in a rather superior way, gives them to the doctor to do something with. He then watches with disdain while the doctor, who seems to fall for this surprisingly readily, works away with mounting exasperation, trying everything he knows. In so doing he experiences more and more of the patient's helpless anxiety. Eventually he cannot stand it any longer. There is a sudden switching of the see-saw and an abrupt reversal, with the doctor suddenly releasing his feelings through sarcasm. The patient crashes down. The doctor feels rather sorry and restores the balance a bit with a physical examination before they part. Within this see-saw relationship there has been a powerful reversal fantasy. The patient has behaved as though he is on one side, appearing exaggeratedly humble and helpless, while seeing the doctor, on the other side, as powerful and mighty. This view is communicated with an irritating irony which seems to say that really the opposite is the truth: the doctor's efforts are laughable while the patient is above it all. The sudden release of feeling in the doctor was one kind of important moment but more important, the echo was still heard a month later when the theme re-emerged. The doctor was sufficiently in tune this time. He was more watchful and less angry. The doctor, instead of anxiously playing along with the patient as he has done previously, admits that the patient has often made him feel rather helpless. It is this sudden spoken thought of what the patient may have wished for some time that is too much for him. The brake is off. Pleasurable disbelief breaks out. There is an important moment shared. They are able to hold the balance for a while in a more even and realistic position. There is greater warmth and a greater area of exchange between the two.

We often discussed the difference between a change in the doctor–patient relationship and a change in the patient's world outside. Clearly it is the latter that is usually the aim of a doctor's work. It is easier to observe changes in the relationship; through the atmosphere of the consultation, the doctor's feelings, the symptoms that the patient brings or the frequency of contact. We were always less certain about how these changes were reflected in whatever changed in the patient's general life. There were always other factors which could have influenced things. But maybe there is more connection than we often observe or admit. In this case there seems to have been a change in the doctor–patient relationship, but what sort of change? How long will it last? And will it help lead to any other change in the patient's life?

The first follow-up interview occurred at the doctor's request, just a week later. The patient reported a complete improvement of his symptoms. The next one happened about six weeks later on the patient's initiative.

This time the patient came to get a prescription for more drops for his iritis and said everything continued to be fine and he had no idea what caused his previous pain. He put me on the spot with some medical questions which I answered a bit uneasily and felt he was playing the exaggerated patient, and me being cautious, you know, just answering questions. He said he had begun thinking a bit about changing his job, he'd made some steps in going to see a careers adviser. And said something about microphones, a radio, working with radio. It turned out he does research for radio programmes. 'But not in front of a microphone,' he said, in a very typical self-disparaging way, 'I wouldn't dream of doing that, oh no, not me.' We talked a bit about his need to be self-disparaging and fear of failure. He left with exaggerated respect, shutting my door over-carefully, leaving me feeling it was shut with irony rather than consideration. This left me feeling, in terms of the sort of interaction we had, nothing much had changed.

The group felt more confident than the doctor who rather irritated them with his pessimism.

'Because there is a change, isn't there? That he's dropped his symptoms.'

'I mean can we relate what happens to what happened in the previous interview? I don't know whether we can or not. But there was a good shaking up, wasn't there?'

'He was in danger of getting an overdose from the doctor, I think.'

'Yes, but this is one where the patient changes but the doctor still doesn't like this guy very much.'

There seems to have been a period of increased intensity, through which the relationship has changed, before settling into a new pattern. We might ask what prevented such a change occurring long before. The ingredients seem to have been there. Why was the relationship held in this rigid and rather unsatisfactory mode for so long? What sometimes releases the doctor? Or, conversely, what holds him back? It often seems that doctors have a distancing device, a back-pedal brake applied to themselves, keeping their patients firmly fixed at a certain distance. The brake reins back the doctor's own feelings, to allow his daily work to proceed. It may be that some strong personal feelings are evoked for him by association with the patient's predicament. Intimacy and engagement of the doctor's feelings have their cost. The interview ends, the patient may take some thoughts away, or allow feelings to surface later, but the doctor has to lose them for the time being and start again with the next patient. Something needs to occur that allows the doctor to relax this inner professional device and release a greater freedom to feel and think and respond with his patient.

One doctor introduced a case by saying, 'Well, I've got a sort of a one, in the sense that I've changed my view of the patient. I'm not sure if the patient's view of herself has in any way become different.'

HANNAH

Well, she's a lady of 71, one of those people who came to this country from Germany in the 1930s. Her husband is her second husband. She's got a couple of kids by her first marriage. I don't know what happened to that. It's also his second marriage. And he's about seven or eight years younger than she is. He's a local businessman and they've both been patients of mine for eight, ten, fifteen years, something like that. And in that time she has had two hip replacements for osteo-arthritis. I've had some medical dealings with her. And then last year, she became depressed and I treated her with good, sound, honest, decent pills (laughs) and, naturally, because she was properly treated she got better. Her husband as I mentioned is younger than she is. I know the son. I don't know the daughter who is older. When I first came into contact with this family some years ago, the son was living at home and I remember that he was a kind of 'yuk', who used to get venereal disease and expect me to forget about that and organize it for him to be attended to. I mean, he really did get up my nose, but to my astonishment he got married and now is a respectable citizen.

Anyway, she came back to see me just before I went away on holiday, feeling depressed, having disturbed sleep, and being upset in the mornings and feeling better as the day wore on. Could she have some more of the tablets? So I gave her some and saw her after a couple of weeks just before I went away and arranged that she would see my partner when I was gone and scaled up the dose of drugs. So she got a bit better and came to see me when I got home again. I have this image of her as a lady who has some physical disability. She's got this osteo-arthritis and she has pills for her depression. And when I was going on holiday we discussed holidays, had a sort of chatting friendly relationship. This time she came she had seen my partner when I was away and she was glad to see me back and she was actually feeling terrible and it was awful. Could she perhaps try not the pills she was having, but the ones she'd had before? I just sort of didn't say very much and said, 'Well, you know, if things are bad, tell me why.' And all of a sudden she said, 'Well, you won't tell anyone.' Then it came out that her husband was having an affair with somebody at work, his secretary or something. She feels it's natural that he should behave like this because she's so much older than he is. He is only sixty-four and they haven't had any sexual relations for some time. Why shouldn't he feel that way and yet she feels it's not fair. And then I said something about 'it must feel very bad to come to this.' And she said, 'what?' And I realized for the very first time that she has a deaf-aid. I suddenly saw her as an old woman with her whole life disappearing and it was something that I just hadn't seen at all. I had grown used to this patient and suddenly there she was, a lonely, desperate, deaf, deprived woman whose husband was deserting her and the children had left home. And all I could see suddenly was her disabilities and her future, or non-future. I suddenly sort of got hit by this tremendous sort of, oh! terrible feeling and guilt that I'd missed it all before. I don't know whether my feeling about her got across the deaf-aid barrier, or what. I don't know what happened. But I do know that it suddenly hit me.

In the doctor's description there seems to be a friendly and rather conscientious aspect to the relationship. He chats about holidays and he carefully arranges for his partner to see the patient while he is away. There is also a feeling that he has held her somewhat at arm's length, perhaps not liking to come into too close contact with her misery, or maybe the memory of her 'awful' son is still active somewhere in his mind as a warning. He does not seem to have been able to let her talk to him before. They have had a 'decent' relationship but a rather distant one. There is a detached irony in some of the description – 'and, naturally, because she was properly treated she got better'. Only a little later on, we are suddenly hit with an awful vision of how this patient is feeling. Rejected and despairing. The doctor is stunned. He suddenly sees her as 'a lonely, desperate, deaf, deprived woman whose husband is deserting her and whose children have left home'. He is shocked. He concludes the interview but was probably hardly able to think after the impact of such a moment.

The patient seems to have had the habit of behaving well for the doctor in rather the same way as she makes herself younger for her husband. We know that often she finds herself to blame when other people reject her. 'It's natural that he should behave like this, because I'm so much older. It's reasonable.' But when she comes for this interview, her feeling of unfairness is closer to the surface than usual. She tells the doctor of her husband's interest in another woman and that she's been feeling awful and is glad to have the doctor back. It seems that the doctor's absence on top of what she was feeling already is too much. She can bear it no longer.

Up to this moment, the doctor seems to have been cruising in quite a relaxed fashion. He responds as he might often in a similar situation, by inviting the patient to tell him why she is feeling terrible and then voices his reaction to what she says, 'It must feel very bad to come to this.' His remark, intended with empathy, only strikes a deafened 'What?' It is then that the true impact of her situation and his reaction to it, hits him. The brake he has applied in his previous dealings with the patient is a little looser this time, and he allows enough of the patient's experience into his own to produce a sudden change. It is as though the doctor has had an image of this patient that he has not wanted to change and which she may have preferred him to have of herself. Suddenly it isn't sufficient for either of them. A further aspect of the reality of their relationship breaks through.

In this case there has been a dramatic change in the doctor's perception. But what effect, if any, does this have on the patient? Or on their relationship together?

'What's interesting is that the important moment was the doctor's shock, not the patient telling you about her miseries although that's important. So what is the effect of the doctor's shock on the patient, it seems to me that this really is the question.'

'This could happen with any patient. You think they are horrible but suddenly you see them differently and you do this visually. This is what we are talking about all the time.'

'But do we assume that it's got to be a mutual thing for it to be effective, that's the question.'

'This is why I brought it up. It seems to me that there's quite a real situation where she may have perceived absolutely nothing, and yet I'm quite certain that the way I will see her in the future will be different.'

The patient returned to see the doctor a month later and was very depressed.

She came back a month later to say she wouldn't be seeing me for a month because she and her husband were going on a business trip. And she wanted to talk to me first. She told me that she was depressed and afraid the pills I had given her were quite useless. She was terrified that she was going to spoil things. What had happened was that her husband and his girlfriend had decided that they must break it off. He was now being very careful and good with her and she was scared that she was going to wreck the prospect of remaking their relationship on the trip, because she was so down and awful. And she said it was terrible, if it really was the affair of his life, it was awful that she should ruin it for him, but on the other hand when they originally got engaged, because of their age difference, she pointed out that perhaps they shouldn't. Tears came into her eyes as she recalled how he had persuaded her after a long interval that they ought to live together and get married. Since the girlfriend has been shed, she said that it's very difficult. He does everything right but he doesn't even want to touch her. He won't even kiss her and certainly they have no sex. I previously thought that sex had finished, but I am wrong; apparently once the hip surgery had been dealt with, they had resumed normal marital relationships until this affair cropped up. But he isn't considerate: he does everything right, but it's not genuine. It's not real. And he has to force himself to do the right thing. And she feels how phony it is and she says, 'how can I, an old woman like me, cope with trying to remake a love affair with him? I love him still, but he doesn't love me and it's terrible.' So I said, 'You must be very cross with him for letting you down like this?' And she said: 'I am not cross with him. It's me, I'm a nuisance. How can I blame him for falling in love with a younger woman?' I felt very strongly the feeling that the insight that I had had was entirely legitimate. That my insight didn't coincide in time with hers. She had had that kind of insight when she discovered about the affair and I picked it up and it was right. So what we were talking about wasn't the angry feelings that she has, but her desperation at falling apart. 'I can't tell you how I feel, I lose the words.' 'What do you mean?' She has a thick German accent, and said: 'I can't remember the words in English and I can't even remember them in German.' And we agreed that she comes and sees me when she comes back from this trip and she's gone off with considerable trepidation as to how the relationship is going to work.

The patient shows herself to be more obviously depressed with the doctor this time. There is less politeness and instead of pretending that the doctor's pills have helped, she straightaway tells him they are useless. She is feeling miserable, but is too depressed to be angry and instead blames herself – 'It's me, I'm a nuisance.' She fears she will spoil things. The awfulness of the vision is verbalized this time. The doctor has steadied his balance. The patient's view isn't changed, but she has a doctor who has adjusted *his* hearing-aid. Whereas previously the doctor–patient relationship seemed to mirror some of the difficulties with her husband: the doctor was polite but distant, not really wanting to 'touch' the patient, and she seemed to hold herself in for the doctor, for fear of spoiling things; now they do so less. The patient seems more confident of not being rejected, and the doctor can allow himself to listen better to her deeper and more unhappy feelings.

In this kind of work, the 'moments of change' are the moments of increased contact between the patient and the doctor; when something important about how the patient is feeling is suddenly felt by the doctor as well. This can change the doctor's whole view of the patient, and the way they respond to each other. These effects may persist for some time and the relationship become more useful to the patient as a result.

7
'Why don't you listen to me, for a change?'

Marie Campkin

'I started with a brief diatribe about smoking. She emerged in the discussion as angry and frustrated with everyone.'

'She asked if she could be referred for manipulation. This was a cue for the doctor to launch into a homily ... that she should take responsibility for helping to bring about her own improved health.'

'For the fourth time I tried to get her to reduce her medication (tranquillizers, etc.) with limited success.'

'The doctor reluctantly decided to broach the subject of his drinking problem. "Is there any point in us talking about this again?" '

(excerpts from the group discussion)

The doctor always has his ready-made refuge of 'respectable medical activities' if he doesn't want to hear what the patient is trying to say. In the past the opportunities for preventive care and patient education have probably been neglected, but there is a danger that in the current fashionable enthusiasm to make good the deficit, doctors may unwittingly let their good intentions get in the way of the patient's present needs.

It is all too easy for the doctor to let his personal objectives pre-empt some of the consultation's content at the expense of the patient's own agenda. These objectives may involve worthy matters such as collecting extra data to improve records, the rationalization of prescribing, a screening exercise such as routine blood pressure checking or some more specifically health-promoting activity such as trying to influence the patient's smoking or drinking habits. But he must not lose sight of the patient's needs by subordinating them to his own interests. In several of our reported cases the doctor had found himself lecturing the patient 'for his own good' – but it was only when he recognized this and desisted that the patient could then make himself heard.

In the case of Alison (described in Chapter 2), after several previous inconclusive interviews the patient had arrived on a busy Monday morning with a new complaint of sore eyes. The doctor discovered, perhaps with relief, that she smoked twenty cigarettes a day, so giving him an excuse to attack her smoking habits (which might even have been marginally relevant to her complaint) rather than to continue his frustrating exploration of her numerous symptoms. But when he began to feel it was becoming a 'nothing' interview, he 'just shut up a bit and she then started talking about how angry she felt'.

Such a retreat into the 'doctor's agenda' may be a sign that he is bored or nonplussed by the problem the patient is presenting and wishes to change the subject; or that he feels threatened by, or unable to deal with the patient's distress and would prefer to re-establish his authority on safer territory. Unfortunately it can be a fertile ground for doctors to display some of their least lovable attributes – self-righteousness, contempt, and condescension – especially when dealing with a patient's weakness which they do not happen to share. No doubt this is why self-help groups are often much more successful than doctors in helping patients with problems such as obesity and alcohol abuse, since these groups usually consist only of people who have experienced and are trying to overcome the same problem themselves.

The following case is one in which the doctor took the initiative in trying to 'educate' the patient.

MARILYN

This 25-year-old Australian girl was shortly leaving to complete her world tour and return home. She had been treated previously for vaginal thrush and had a recurrence for which she wanted further treatment. Meanwhile she had developed some pains and asked my advice on whether she ought to have some manipulative treatment. I wasn't very receptive to this idea. I could see her half-turned towards me and she seemed to be sprawled on the chair and overweight. I became very didactic and told her that in my opinion she was seeking to be put right by things that other people would do for her. In other words, she would achieve more, health-wise, if she got some of her weight down. This was a rather negative, antagonistic, and paternalistic approach which I think was right and honest. The interesting thing was that this must have connected with something in her, and she said, 'Yes, you're quite right.'

The group thought that the doctor had been rather unkind in ignoring her symptoms and then adding insult to injury with a verbal assault. It was a 'manipulation' of a sort, though not of the kind she was asking for. Yet the patient seemed to be reasonably satisfied with this outcome – perhaps she felt that the doctor was at least expressing some concern for her. The doctor said that he felt that she was trying to get something more out of the National Health Service before leaving the country. This, together with his perception of her plumpness, equated in his mind with self-indulgence. In retrospect he agreed with some of the group's criticism of his approach.

I saw her again two weeks later, as she was getting an inoculation from the nurse before her departure. This time I noticed a pleasant red-head, not all that fat. She announced with a laugh that she had not lost any weight. I then acceded to her request for a repeat prescription of her oral contraceptive by giving her six months' supply without demur, despite my previous strictures about her getting all she could from the National Health Service. Perhaps this was my turn to be the subject of manipulation!

If this relationship had continued longer the doctor might have been able to find out what Marilyn really needed. Certainly these rather superficial transactions shed little light on that question.

In contrast, the doctor may feel he has a good idea of what the patient is needing, but somehow the 'health education' aspect can become a collusive activity between the doctor and patient, providing a legitimate area of mutual concern while tacitly by-passing some much more uncomfortable subject-matter. The doctor may be a reluctant partner in this conspiracy and want to take the initiative by breaking out of the trap. On the other hand he must also learn the importance of sometimes respecting the patient's ideas above his own.

NICOLA

This is a girl of 23. This particular interview was the sixth or seventh. When she came to see me she said she had a weight problem and wanted to know how she could lose some weight, from 9½ stone back to 8 stone as she had been previously.

When the doctor looked through her notes he was reminded that she had major congenital abnormalities – an absent uterus, vaginal septum, and only one kidney. And yet all this seems to have been put right at the back of her mind and the thing that preoccupies her is how to lose weight. At 9½ stone she is plump but by no means unattractive, and no-one would guess there is anything wrong with her female apparatus.

She gave me the opportunity to ask because she was worried about only having one kidney and wanted to know which side it was on. So I said, 'there are other things wrong as well,' and I asked about boyfriends and she had had one with whom some sort of sexual activity had taken place – but they had now broken off. At the moment she hadn't got a steady boyfriend.

The doctor was anxious to help and eager to offer advice and to make enquiries about the possibilities of plastic surgery for her. But 'she didn't want to have anything more to do with the hospital, and please could I help her with her weight.' The doctor agreed to supervise her and gave her a diet. As he said, 'I decided if I didn't want to lose her, I had better keep the dialogue going in some way, even if it was only to do with weight.'

Subsequent interviews were indeed occupied with talk of calories and metabolism, and little else. It seemed it was bearable for her to talk about her weight, or even her missing kidney, but not about the implications of her other defects. At one point, Nicola's father visited the doctor to express anxiety because she seemed disproportionately worried about her weight and was now refusing to go to work or out of the house until she got down to 8 stone.

The group found it puzzling that the family's concern seemed to be of such recent origin. The diagnosis had only been made when she was twenty-one, eighteen months ago, despite the primary amenorrhoea which must have been a growing worry to her from her mid-teens onwards.

Other information which the doctor later recalled was that a younger sister had been anorexic for a while, and the patient herself, whose disgust at her weight and unwillingness to go out seemed suggestive of anorexia, had in fact only achieved her 'best weight' of 8 stone by induced vomiting and laxative abuse. This had occurred about a year after the diagnosis of her congenital abnormalities was made. At that time the doctor had managed to dissuade her from using such extreme methods of slimming and her weight had promptly gone back to 9½ stone.

The doctor formulated this working diagnosis: 'Her feelings about her abnormalities are more than she can bear. They remain hidden from her and instead she has determined to coerce her body into a different, more slender shape. The dread of being recognized, or of recognizing herself, as a freak, makes her hide herself at home. She appreciates the fact that I am taking an interest in her, but wishes to remain in control of the agenda.'

At the next interview, three weeks later, the doctor noticed she looked fatter, and her weight had in fact risen to 10 stone. However, she said she had been having acupuncture treatment which was very successful. It doesn't make her lose weight, but it is making her more comfortable with the idea of herself as a fatter girl and she was now able to go out of the house more easily.

'Now I can come and see you whenever you like,' she said. The doctor was hurt by her defection and piqued that the acupuncturist seemed to have succeeded where he had failed and he did not recognize that this remark could be a request for more of his attention. He casually suggested she could return in a month or so.

The doctor's conclusion, after the group had discussed this interview, was that he had been relieved of the task of making her slim, and may be given another task, but so far had not found out what it was to be.

When Balint likened the doctor to a 'drug', he insisted that the doctor's use of himself should become as conscious and considered an act as the issuing of a prescription, with due regard to frequency, dosage, and possible side-effects. It may be that we should regard 'health advice' as another kind of prescription. Statistics purporting to state, for example, how many patients could be induced to stop smoking if the general practitioner routinely followed certain procedures give no indication of the possible hidden costs of this activity.

If we are using ourselves and our influence to persuade patients to make difficult changes in their life-styles, we owe it to them to be fully aware of the significance of what we are doing and its possible consequences.

No doubt there are many patients who can accept some general suggestions about their eating, drinking, or smoking habits. Indeed they may request them or at least recognize their relevance to their medical problems. But the equilibrium of patients' lives may be finely balanced between the various stresses caused by illness, anxiety, marital, social, and financial problems on the one side, and such 'crutches' as alcohol, tobacco, food, and tranquillizers on the other. We must not underestimate the effect of depriving them of one or more of these sources of support. Sometimes we must be ready to admit that continuation of the 'bad habit' may, for the time being, be preferable to the side-effects of its immediate cessation. And when it is necessary to insist on the patient's compliance, we must also be prepared to provide real support ourselves in adequate frequency and dosage.

VIVIENNE
When I first joined the practice twenty years before, I used to visit

Vivienne's father, who was housebound due to chronic lung disease. Vivienne was then aged 18, and was soon married and had had a child, when at the age of 21, she began to develop severe agoraphobia. She ran the gamut of treatment over the next six years: drugs, psychotherapy, behavioural therapy, and four months as an in-patient, eventually ending up on heavy doses of drugs from yet another hospital. From 1972 this medication was continued within the practice, the patient attending frequently with various anxiety symptoms and seeing other doctors.

I had initiated her referrals in the first place, but during this period I hardly saw her. When I did, my abiding impression was of her zombie-like appearance and manner, a combination of drugged behaviour and weird eye make-up. By this time she had had two brief marriages and was co-habiting with her latest boyfriend. She had also developed a drinking problem. In 1974 and 1978 she had two more sons, who were apparently none the worse for her drink- and drug-taking throughout the pregnancies.

In 1979 she had a home visit from a brash Australian trainee, who told her bluntly that she should 'take a look at herself, sitting amongst her fags, booze, and pills'. This made a great impression on her and seems to have been a turning-point. He saw her several times and got her off barbiturates, but she was still drinking and taking an assortment of antidepressants, tranquillizers, and sleeping pills.

One interesting sequel was that her annual surgery attendance rate dropped from over thirty in 1979 to single figures within the next two years, and some time later she stopped herself drinking, though she continued with her repeat prescriptions.

Sometime in 1981 she drifted back into my care with various medical problems, and I made several attempts to get her to reduce her medication, without much success.

On the fourth occasion, while treating her for phlebitis, I had a further discussion with her and suggested she should now take the tablets when she felt she needed them, rather than routinely, and keep a record of how many she took each day.

A month later she returned for a further consultation about her persistent phlebitis, and handed over a small notebook in which she had recorded, not just her medication, but a moving day-to-day account of her life and feelings.

After she had left I read the diary and realized for the first time how very difficult her life seemed to be, fighting against phobic symptoms, anxious about her children's behaviour and her reaction to it, and intermittently depressed and hopeless.

She had taken up my casual suggestion to note her drug-taking, but had chosen to interpret it in the wider sense of recording her life and the effect of the drugs on her. This communication of herself and her distress compelled me to become more conscious of her as an individual and not as an exercise in the reduction of psychotropic drug-taking.

The patient volunteered that she felt more alive on fewer drugs, and for the first time in years had been able to make some important decisions about her life, including realizing that a proposed reunion with her separated common-law husband would be a disaster. She feels that in order to live with him again she would have to be permanently doped and drugged and would soon be looking at life again through the bottom of a vodka bottle.

On the same day that she handed over the notebook, Vivienne rode on a bus for the first time in twelve years. Within the next few weeks she had a minor operation in hospital without falling to pieces, and survived a 30-mile minicab journey to take her children to spend Christmas with her mother.

Her relationship with me became much more relaxed, with Vivienne herself having taken over the task of dealing with her medication, to such good effect that she virtually discontinued all her drugs over the next six months, apart from new treatment for pre-menstrual tension, which the diary had revealed as a considerable factor contributing to her problems. There were fairly frequent supportive interviews and I came to appreciate the self-deprecating sense of humour which seemed to tide Vivienne over her blackest moments.

A crisis arose when she suddenly discovered that her mother had advanced cancer. She was unable to visit her, because she was in a distant hospital and all forms of travelling still presented great difficulties. Within a few weeks her mother died and Vivienne was in considerable distress. There were several interviews which began, 'I don't think I can cope any more', but ended with a rueful acceptance that life would go on. She went back onto sleeping tablets for a while without any misgivings on her part or mine about giving them up again when the time was right.

Having acquired a drug dependency of mainly iatrogenic origin, this patient was subjected to rather contrasting styles of 'health education' to try to remedy the situation. The first, from the Australian trainee, was tough but concerned, and perhaps the more effective for coming from an attractive man of her own age. Certainly this particular form of 'shock treatment' would not have been in the repertoire of her present doctor, but Vivienne remembers it without resentment and admits it had a profound effect, though it was some time in bearing fruit.

The doctor's own initial efforts were quite ineffective, because they were impersonal – a clinical duty undertaken without real understanding of what was being demanded. As she admitted to the group, 'The way I suppose it started was as a pill-reducing exercise, such as one undertakes on quite a lot of people in a more or less routine fashion. If they are on the pills you try and get them off or cut them down – rather like trying to stop people from smoking without necessarily wanting to get too involved as to why they do it.'

It seems that in this case it was only after the doctor had dropped her attempt to change the patient's habits, that changes began to occur. Once the picture of the patient's life, revealed by the notebook, had shocked the doctor out of her stereotyped behaviour, she could respond with real concern while Vivienne found her own way of dealing with the problem. Thus released from the role of 'health educator' the doctor could even give permission for her to resume her drugs when circumstances changed, without having to regard this as a setback or an admission of defeat.

There are some similarities between this and the story of Ralph (described in Chapter 6) – the 'lonely, homosexual alcoholic' who, when he was allowed to stop talking about drinking, was able to express instead his fears about suffocation and death. Again, the work really began when the focus shifted from the problem to the patient. The doctor's unreal expectations and the patient's meaningless promises could then both be set aside, so that periods of abstinence could be welcomed and setbacks tolerated within a relationship which was no longer dependent on the impossible obligation for one party to cure and the other to conform.

In general practice a good deal of everyday work takes place at the level of treatment of symptoms. This may be acceptable provided the underlying condition is recognized as being minor and self-limiting. Just as we prescribe a decongestant for sinusitis, an analgesic for a sprain, or an antacid for a dietary indiscretion, so we may also discuss smoking, eating, and drinking behaviour in a fairly superficial way with those patients for whom this seems appropriate. But discussing the patient's habits is not a substitute for attempting to get to grips with the underlying distress of which seriously self-destructive behaviour may be the presenting symptom. Nor is assuming an obligation to alter his behaviour an adequate alternative to looking with the patient at his whole life to see how, or indeed whether, he can make some changes.

No matter how strongly he believes that the patient should follow the proffered advice, a doctor must always be ready to hear the patient's reasons for being unable or unwilling to comply. In this way he may sometimes find a route to a new understanding and tolerance of the patient's life and problems. Fruitless repetition of argument and admonition can reduce the whole relationship to a stalemate. The patient might become reluctant even to present with new and possibly important symptoms for fear of further scolding, or out of guilt that as they must be of his own making he has no right to complain. What price health education then?

8
Being there
Paul Julian

We all have an inborn facility to heal ourselves. Our own flesh heals without our conscious instruction. With the high expectations of today's technological and scientific world this tends to be forgotten. All modern 'talking treatments' aim to restore this innate ability and to help patients switch on their own healing facility. One aim of Balint training is to enable general practitioners to help patients mobilize their own resources. For a doctor to be effective in this sort of work, he should feel free enough to be as responsive as possible to his patient.

It is proposed to call this kind of open availability 'being there'. This phrase needs clarification as unfortunately it can have two almost opposite meanings. It could be understood to imply continuity: being there when needed. This is a description of the long-term context of general practice. However, it is the other sense that is intended here: 'being present', the doctor giving the patient his complete attention. It describes a quality of the contact and not its quantity; the intensity of the doctor's concentration and understanding of what is happening at that moment. Being truly 'there' and nowhere else. It can be difficult to shift into the 'here and now' of the consultation, but making this change has a significant bearing on how the doctor perceives and responds to his patient.

Both doctor and patient tend to be readily deflected from being fully aware of what is actually happening in the consultation. For instance, the doctor's perception of a well-known patient can easily be fixed in the past. Much of the work of general practice involves caring for people over a long period of time and most doctors have at some time stumbled into a diagnosis of, say, myxoedema or Parkinsonism which, because of their familiarity with the patient, had previously gone unnoticed. Familiarity can be a trap.

A doctor may find it easier to be aware of what is happening when dealing with a pressing physical problem like an acute attack of asthma or heart failure. Doctors are taught to recognize such illness. Emotional crises are more complex and the doctor's own feelings become more involved. In perceiving internal changes, the signs the doctor elicits are not externally measurable. They depend on his own responses in a fundamental way, for they involve his personal emotional reactions to the patient. One doctor's degree of irritation or attraction to a patient will differ from another's as will his perceptions and blind spots.

There has been emphasis in recent years, when studying consultations, on finding out 'why the patient came today?' – a legitimate question which focuses the doctor's attention on the present. However, the question 'why?' still has prime position and can become a distracting preoccupation if the doctor then feels compelled to prise this information from the patient. It is preferable if the patient simply feels able to tell him. The difficulty may lie as much in the doctor who will not allow the patient to talk as in the patient who seems reluctant to do so.

When a doctor wants to understand why an acute attack of asthma or heart failure has occurred, he often questions the patient with the legitimate assumption that he knows more about the disease and how it may have arisen than the patient does himself. If he makes the same assumption about the patient's emotional world he gets stuck, for the patient knows far more than the doctor and cause and effect are idiosyncratic. Accordingly, asking the question 'why?' may be inappropriate in these circumstances, for the patient may either be unaware of the answer, or in possession of it but unable or unwilling to talk. Focusing on 'how?' the patient is behaving may be more helpful.

Even simple observations about the present can also be distorted by anxiety about the future. If the future looks bleak or empty or the patient appears stuck in a rut, the doctor's own feelings of hopelessness or impotence may overwhelm him and lead him to feel driven 'to do' things for the patient, instead of 'being there' to understand. The doctor may be under such pressure that he confuses his own needs with the patient's. 'You're a nice case of Diazepam, you'd better have some anxiety,' describes the doctor's need to do something and his inability to stay with the patient. If strong urges like this can be perceived by the doctor as part of the patient's world, he may be able to tolerate them better.

The doctor's usefulness in this sort of therapy depends on the sense he makes of his perceptions and how he uses them; whilst sustaining accurate attention and responding to the patient appropriately.

To show how 'being there' can contribute to helping patients, two cases will be described. In the first the doctor seems to have freedom to explore things with his patient, although it is obvious that this had not always been so.

SARAH

She was a rather large, overbearing, elderly woman, attending frequently for supervision of her hypertension and late-onset asthma. At first the doctor had felt overwhelmed and had kept her at a distance, but he had warmed to her a little as he came to see her as a lonely widow whose idealized only daughter seemed too busy to visit her.

One day she came for a 'routine' consultation – a blood pressure check and repeat prescription. Lulled by the familiarity of the situation, the doctor was 'coasting along, thinking with relief that it would be a quick interview,' when she mentioned that her daughter was expecting a baby very soon. His automatic response with 'appropriate' expressions of pleasure and satisfaction was suddenly cut short by the realization that she was in fact furious and critical, complaining that the pregnancy was 'too late' and her daughter unprepared.

Struck by the disparity between his assumptions and her feelings, the doctor now began to concentrate while the patient reminded him, with much emotion, that her daughter was adopted as she had been unable to conceive because of an abnormal (bicornuate) uterus. The daughter's casual announcement that she had become pregnant 'by mistake' was clearly in unforgivable contrast to her own years of fruitless and humiliating investigations for infertility.

The whole consultation had changed from a straightforward repeat performance to a highly charged communication, giving the doctor a totally new view of the patient. His working diagnosis now became 'a woman who has always felt herself a freak, with strong feelings of failure and dissatisfaction with herself as a wife and mother, facing powerful and confusing feelings in relation to her adopted daughter having a baby.'

While presenting the case to the group the doctor recalled that the daughter's pregnancy had in fact been mentioned in passing during an earlier consultation. Sarah had also requested referral to an asthma specialist, so that she could be admitted to hospital if the need should arise in future. The possibility of a significant connection between these two circumstances had escaped him at the time and he had forgotten about it until later.

The doctor had been coasting along, ready to repeat the previous medication and make light conversation. He had forgotten that his patient's daughter was pregnant and he seems to have been a long way off. But perhaps there was more to it than that. He seems to have been quite unconsciously provoking the patient by not understanding her properly. He had after all known the details of her past history and had been told that her daughter was pregnant, but he had forgotten both these important facts. Did his behaviour perhaps mirror in some way the provocation she had made him feel in the past? He certainly had to recover quickly and come back to be with his patient and her present troubled feelings. He was free enough to do so because, although she was a frequent attender and exacting, she had become much more tolerable over the last few months. In this consultation she suddenly became alive and more real for the doctor. Tolerability shifted into acceptance and this allowed the interview to open up.

The group's discussion of the case centred round the question 'What was she so angry about?' Was it resentment that her daughter had achieved, effortlessly and almost by accident, the pregnancy that she herself was denied? She must have been about the same age when she had given up hope and resorted to adoption. Was it distress at the daughter's casual, almost indifferent attitude to the pregnancy, carelessly declining the pleasures of anticipation and preparation which the patient had not been able to enjoy? Was it apprehension lest her daughter might fail as a mother as she may have felt herself to have done? Or fear that she will have no part in this baby who is, and yet is not, her only grandchild?

It was still unclear what she was asking from her doctor. He had now 'heard' what she was trying to tell him. Would that be sufficient, or would she go on to become 'ill', having prepared the way for herself by engineering the specialist referral? Perhaps her existing illnesses – asthma and hypertension – should now be reconsidered in the light of the tensions in her life implicit in these revelations. The interview had such a profound effect on the doctor that it was interesting to wonder whether the patient had been equally affected by it, or whether the next time would revert to 'business as usual.'

Shortly after there was a phone call about some blood tests, and a consultation a few days later began with a series of physical complaints, while the doctor wondered whether to play along or to try and steer her back to the subject of her daughter. Eventually she did refer to it and she and the doctor became 'like a couple of grannies' as she gave an account of the baby's birth and of her anxiety that her daughter might become depressed and reject the baby. She also shared with him the secret of an intimate moment of mingled triumph and pain when a relative, unaware of her daughter's adoption, said the baby resembled her.

After a sticky start, this case seems to have been a success, for despite all the patient's physical needs and strong anxieties, the patient had been able to use the doctor. She had retained her independence. He had moved quickly to be with her when needed and reacted attentively when she had shared her feelings with him. He may have been the only person with whom she could safely talk in this way.

PEGGY

Peggy is a housewife. She's aged 33 and her husband is aged 50. They have one boy aged 5 and a girl of 18 months and she has been on the doctor's list since the baby was born. She suffered from migraine and had first been seen when the baby was five days old. The doctor had been called to see her that night as he was on duty and found that she had an infected perineum. She was obviously in great pain and had a temperature, but was carrying on bravely. She had a boyish hair cut and seemed a jolly sort of athletic person, so the doctor coped with her in the same sort of way, efficient and smiling. Large doses of antibiotics were prescribed and she made a good recovery. In the next few months she saw several doctors in the practice for a number of routine matters, then consulted about the children. The doctor carried on in the same jolly way with her as this seemed to be how she behaved. The latest consultation was about her migraine. She had two severe attacks, one a year previously and one a week ago. The discussion turned on the stress of having two young children and she said, 'Ah well, the first one last year, yes. My mother-in-law was on the phone and the children were playing up and that was an awful time, so I can understand that. But the second time, oh no, certainly not. Everything was fine. It was Friday evening and my husband had come in from work and the children were playing happily, so it can't be emotional.' The doctor accepted this and discussed the possibility that chocolate or cheese or eye-strain might be causative factors, but he was getting nowhere and feeling more uncomfortable. He felt that he couldn't get through to the patient in spite of trying, so prescribed some pills for the next time. She then said, 'I'm scared it might happen when there's nobody around to help me with the children. It would be really frightening.' The doctor suddenly found himself replying, 'Well, it won't, migraines never happen when you can't have them.' And she said, 'That's interesting. In fact, the first time my husband was home and the second time too. He had just walked in the door so it was quite true. Well having children is of course rather a stress, isn't it?' She was intrigued by the idea, accepted that it seemed to be true for her, took her prescription and walked out. The doctor felt that he had broken through and made real contact; had reached her feelings about how awful it could be to have to look after two kids.

In the discussion it became clear that the doctor had not just handed out reassurance. He felt that he had shared a moment with the patient about the strain of looking after the children. But had it really been shared? The patient had said, 'I'm really scared it might happen when there's nobody around.' It was after this that the doctor found himself responding so positively and with such inexplicable conviction. He consciously heard her say how hard it was to look after the children, but he seems to have responded to her fear that she might explode out of control into migraine while looking after the children *alone*. Perhaps it was this, her fear of losing control, that the doctor had reached by his own rather uncontrolled and spontaneous remark. The causes of her anxieties, whether they were connected to the stresses of bringing up children or not, seem less important than the doctor getting through to her that he understood something of the necessity for her to keep potentially explosive anxieties bottled up. He allowed her to realize that for her, migraines were a communication which had no point unless someone was there to receive them. They wouldn't occur (or she wouldn't allow them to occur) on her own.

It was clear that the interview had been lively. Indeed this liveliness resonated between the doctor and the patient. Like the first case, this doctor had intuitively chosen a mode of communication that the patient used and understood. On the surface it was kept brisk and cheerful, like the patient herself, but seems to have been completely in accord with the patient's need for both reassurance and self-understanding. Three years later he reviewed the case.

She brought her four-year-old to the Well Baby clinic recently. 'We met when she was born, doctor,' she reminded him. She had had only two very slight migraines since the earlier discussion. She remains a jolly sporty type and wanted nothing further for herself, just to use the general practitioner in an ordinary way for the family.

The doctor felt that the patient did not want him to get inside her fears, but rather to 'storm me into becoming a kindly caring man who would allay these fears whenever necessary.' But for one significant moment he had been able to respond to her with immediacy and presence. They had a moment of understanding and accord when she had allowed her fears, albeit briefly, to show through.

It will have become evident that, although this way of working with patients requires a different discipline than that involved in offering help through long interviews, it is still mediated through the same currency, the doctor's feelings. It is hoped that the description of these cases will have shown the importance and some of the problems for the doctor in sustaining himself in the present with his patient; and allowing himself freedom to react with spontaneity to the patient's barely perceived needs. It is not a technique, more a frame of mind for allowing a contact to spark up between the patient and his doctor. This, it is hoped, will rekindle the patient's awareness of some inner part of himself and lead him on towards the process of healing.

9
The dependent patient
Cyril Gill

Important moments of shared understanding are both the means by which a relationship is built up and also the means by which the patient uses it. Some may use this relationship well and others may show little change but remain dependent on the doctor. The relationship may have many shades of feeling for a patient. For example, the doctor may be seen as having echoes of a parent or a potential lover perhaps, safely defused by the clear understanding of the limits of the doctor–patient relationship. Any relevant problems in relating to people may well be enacted between doctor and patient.

'Help me, but don't get too close' is a crude description of a fairly common way that some patients present, reflecting their problems in relating to everyone including the doctor. They may long for warmth and understanding, but if the doctor gets too close to the heart of the problem they may get frightened or angry. Such people avoid close intimacy, fearing hurt or scorn. Others feel useless, and hide this with an aggressive superiority which is difficult to pierce. Occasionally the patient may be helped to understand such things within the doctor–patient context and learn from it (Stuart in Chapter 6), but more often the patient tries to approach the doctor in different ways and may only learn to keep a safe distance from him and others. At worst, he will learn nothing and spend a lifetime presenting a shifting target of untreatable bodily complaints to different doctors. Everyone knows patients like this who can never be helped. By contrast, the ideal outcome for an interview or series of interviews, is that the patient will learn something useful and not need the doctor any more. Between these two extremes lies the average patient, who gains a little understanding, but remains to some extent dependent on the doctor when things get bad.

Such dependency is readily acceptable if the patient has diabetes or multiple sclerosis, but often doctors are afraid of it when the problems are mainly emotional. This is understandable if the patient is excessively demanding, manipulative, or defeating, but fortunately most are not like that. Such manipulations may decrease if the doctor can understand a little better what the patient wants from him. There are doctors who dislike weak, anxious patients, and others who actually enjoy them. Unfortunately there are many possible gratifications for a doctor, both subtle and crude, apart from the obvious sexual ones. It is not uncommon for a doctor to spend much time and effort acting in a way that gets the approval of certain patients, though he may be horrified when he discovers he is doing so. Patients may say, 'My doctor is so kind and understanding.' If the doctor concerned is actually aiming for this, he will surely fail to help the patient. Doctors are rightly anxious about their part in allowing patients to become dependent on them, in case they are only indulging in a collusive enjoyment of some kind. They need to be aware of what they are trying to do, of what is actually going on, and their therapeutic concern must be paramount. It is, however, true that helping dependent patients is an important part of every doctor's work. Psychiatrists usually dismiss patients whom they cannot help, but general practitioners must be available at short notice for all. The troubled patient may well present with bodily symptoms if he cannot get our attention otherwise. Whether one likes it or not, many patients are dependent, and the problem is to understand this situation and contain it, if it is not possible to help the patient need the doctor less.

There are some people who need to carry someone around in their minds to use when they are under stress and the general practitioner may be used in this way. One patient said, 'I know I don't say much when I am here, but I often talk to you in my head at other times.' This patient can share her feelings with her own image of the doctor, but cannot manage without an occasional visit to top up this support. It is likely that other recurrent attenders with less awareness are attempting to use their doctors in a similar way. Many patients attend with puzzling minor ailments that go away again without any clear reason. Some patients seem to enjoy defeating the doctor, and it is comforting to imagine that perhaps they function better in some way in return for his discomfiture. Such difficult relationships are accepted as part of general practice and all one can do is to aim towards understanding and honesty.

Many elderly patients come to the general practitioner recurrently for a repeat dose of his attention. There is often a regular scenario about these visits. The doctor may be asked to take their blood pressure or listen to their hearts, when medically this is quite unnecessary. Perhaps a parent died of a stroke at a similar age, or they are anxious to be well for some coming event. Often they say they are ready for death, but scared of the process of dying, or that they would prefer a quick death to a lingering one. Behind such obvious fears may be many other things they want to share. Regrets and failures, family matters of all kinds, but often there is also a wish to feel that somebody knows about them, accepts them, and will remember if they are alive or dead. One very healthy old lady said, 'Is it true that you can't sign a death certificate if you haven't seen me for two weeks?' She accepts the idea of death, but does not want strange doctors poking about inside her afterwards. Her respectability reaches as far as the grave. Doctor and patient could laugh about this, but not about the small details of her past life which she has mentioned on occasions, nor the old newspaper cuttings she has shown him. Somehow this shared intimacy about her life gives it validity and presumably she hopes that some memory of her will survive in the doctor's mind after she dies. On occasions such a relationship may be threatened by events.

MISS WATSON

Miss Watson is an elderly lady, well-known to the doctor. He has seen her regularly for fifteen years for the usual minor problems of old age. She is fiercely independent, yet needs help on occasions. Her niece came to live with her and was rather a moaner. She had bronchitis and was reluctant to get up again and look after the old lady who needed her help. The doctor found her rather trying. Unfortunately he missed the fact that she was really quite ill with renal failure. Eventually she was admitted to hospital and died, in spite of transfusions and dialysis. The doctor felt that he had failed to diagnose this serious illness in the niece, and so did the old lady. She summoned him to explain it all. He was absolutely honest, explaining exactly what he had missed, but he also admitted that he had not liked her and this had impaired his judgement. Probably the old lady did not like her much either and this may have helped the situation. Doubtless she was worrying about whether the doctor would miss important illness when it struck her too, but she probably sensed that he liked her a lot more than the niece. The stern old lady melted as she agreed with the general practitioner that her family was difficult. By the end of the interview she had become a frail old lady again. The doctor's failure was forgiven and they had restored their previously comfortable relationship of trust and mutual respect.

A few months later the doctor reported that he had seen her several times for trouble with her hearing-aid and each time she had also talked about minor family difficulties as before. The doctor could have tried to excuse his error by saying that renal failure is easy to miss, or that nothing could have been done anyway, but he instinctively chose honesty, which suited them both much better. Some doctors pretend (with the patient's collusion) that they will keep them alive for ever. There was no nonsense like that here. The old lady could forgive a lapse, even a fatal one, engendered by antipathy, so long as the doctor gets on well with her and cares about the quality of her life.

Another case illustrates the importance of ongoing support, with very slight changes in the patient herself.

ANITA

Anita, aged 37, is the only child of anxious parents. Her mother came from a large family herself, and Anita was always aware that her mother would have liked a large family too. She was overprotected as a child, yet she felt she was expected to shine for both parents and always hid her real feelings from them. She escaped to London, gained a diploma in teaching, then abandoned this for secretarial work. She has severe bouts of depression for which she attends the general practitioner. Antidepressants have little effect. She sits there mutely, hiding her feelings from the general practitioner too, until he encourages her to feel free to talk or cry. She lives in a hostel with several other girls and they are important to her like a family, so she is upset when any of the girls leave. The doctor has become very important to her. She no longer feels she must please him like her parents, though she remains very quiet and passive. She describes her father as anxious and withdrawn, hiding his feelings except when he thinks he is ill. Her mother also hides her feelings and is not very sympathetic to father's imagined ills. When her father had a slight stroke, Anita seemed to improve in spirits, much to the doctor's surprise. She said she could relate to him in a different way when he was really ill and she had now realized that everything that happened to her parents was not her fault.

A year later she set up a flat with a girlfriend and this has been a much more stable arrangement. She is certainly less depressed, but needs to keep in touch with her doctor fairly often. One day she complained of abdominal discomfort and he found a mass. She was admitted to hospital and had a terrifying week of investigations, that eventually revealed a benign cyst which was aspirated and disappeared. The doctor visited her in hospital, where she was tearful and withdrawn. Later she told the doctor that the thought of her parents finding out where she was terrified her more than serious illness itself. She felt guilt and fear at the thought of letting them down with illness. She is aware that these are her own feelings more than her parents'.

The group discussed this case and felt there were many things she was not discussing with her general practitioner. However, it was difficult to reach the origins of her guilt and fear. She slept in her parents' bedroom until she was 9 years old, but was not aware of being in the way. She talks quite freely of the fact that her parents never had any sex life after she was born. Mother thought it was dirty and father would have no say in the matter. Anita gives the doctor the impression that she has no sexual thoughts herself. The doctor feels that she relates to him like a child, and although she has possible homosexual feelings, there is no such relationship to her new flatmate. Though she is undoubtedly better, this is as much due to events as to the doctor's help. She is still working on her problems and trying to understand them and free herself from this bondage to her parents, or her image of them. She is still very dependent on the doctor, who is a token of the more permissive parent she needs.

She is one of many patients who unconsciously try the doctor out to see if he fits their needs. This may lead only to frustration and rejection, and being let down once again, but occasionally the doctor can spot what is happening and help them to see what they are doing.

A psychotherapist would give such patients limited time and attempt to work through the problems in the relationship between them. A family doctor develops a similar relationship, with many brief interactions. The process of 'working through' is usually much less thorough, but the relationship may continue for many years, the general practitioner acting as a replacement for some important person that the patient needs. This will be an idealized image projected onto the doctor, who will probably be quite a different person in real life. For those who cannot grow away from this dependency, the doctor may have to remain an important person indefinitely.

10
Travelling hopefully
John Salinsky

As doctors we are naturally very concerned about the outcome of our work. It is important to know whether the treatment has been successful and the patient cured or at least relieved of some of his symptoms. But the assessment of outcome can be very difficult even where purely physical disorders are concerned: witness the large and complicated clinical trials which are needed before we can decide whether a new drug for arthritis or hypertension is any better than its predecessors. When we try to evaluate the effects of psychological forms of treatment, the problems become formidable. In this book we have been discussing not just 'a disease' or 'a treatment regime', but a sort of therapeutic philosophy applied to a diverse collection of people with all kinds of problems expressed both physically and emotionally.

We are likely to be told that as our ideas are not susceptible to validation they cannot be put forward as a contribution to science and are to be regarded as articles of belief or even faith. Since we like to think of ourselves as practising a science as well as an art, this verdict seems unacceptable. Surely we can find examples of patients who have improved considerably under our care? But can we relate the 'improvement' we see to the work we have been doing? What criteria can we find to measure the outcome of a doctor–patient relationship? We might hope to 'enable the patient to realize more of his potential' but could reasonably be asked to define what we meant by that. We might then decide to follow up our patient's progress by an assessment of his achievements in a number of areas generally agreed to be important in the fulfilment of potential. Does he have a happy marriage? Has he been successful in his career? Does he have a low score on a questionnaire designed to elicit 'neurotic symptoms'? Does he take tranquillizers? Unfortunately life has many ups and downs, with or without the interventions of a family doctor. A lot might depend on the year, or even the day on which the evaluation was carried out. Even when a patient really seems to have changed remarkably for the better, we remain uncertain as to how much is due to the doctor's influence and how much to outside factors totally beyond his control or outside his knowledge.

It is my belief that attempts to measure outcome as a way of validating our work are neither profitable nor necessary. We would do better, as was mentioned in the introduction, to see ourselves as natural historians writing descriptions, rather than experimental scientists making predictions and then testing them against a null hypothesis. However, there is a further problem in that the natural historian doctor may observe the behaviour of his subject, but can only infer what he is thinking and feeling. In the case reports in this book, the reporting doctors have tried to make perceptive guesses about the effects on their patients of interviews which the doctors saw as significant. But they were only guesses.

We do not really know what the patients experienced during these consultations because we cannot ask them and on the whole they do not tell us. On the other hand, we know a great deal about what the doctors experienced and I think this is worth examining more closely.

Let us look again at some of the cases in earlier chapters, and the way the doctors describe their own feelings about their patients. Here is Ralph's doctor from Chapter 6:

'I know him to be a longstanding alcoholic . . . I haven't had many contacts with him, but those I have had have been discouraging . . . so really I was quite prepared to treat his cough and not do anything very much else . . . I sort of did the ritual examination of his chest . . . and for some reason I decided that perhaps . . . one should, once again talk about this drinking.'

Initially then, the doctor is fairly unenchanted by her patient and is about to rubber stamp his chest with her stethoscope, when something prompts her, wearily but dutifully, to mention 'this drinking'. A little later on, her feelings about him are quite different: 'At some point I was beginning to feel more sympathetic to him . . . I was hoping I was talking in terms of seeing him again on Monday or Tuesday to try and keep hold of him.' And finally: 'He went off looking quite cheerful and I felt quite cheerful . . . as he went out I felt a bit hopeful about him.'

After the next interview, the doctor is much less hopeful about Ralph's prognosis as an alcoholic, but has become much more interested in his fears about death and suffocation. She has started to feel responsible for him while realizing that the work is going to be more like terminal care than rehabilitation.

Stuart (see Chapter 6) is a young man whose doctor at first finds him 'irritating and unexpressive'. We are told about 'various physical symptoms . . . incredibly boring and very, very detailed, terribly distant, a very controlled sort of aggression.' A little later on: 'I felt really furious with him and actually gave him . . . a good sort of bashing.'

The interview is subsequently described as 'a kick up the backside' which the doctor has delivered, albeit only verbally, but with a certain relish. He is angry with the patient for being so 'superior and disdainful' and with himself for having treated him so respectfully in the past. A little further on he finds himself telling the patient that he has found him powerful and intimidating; Stuart appears stunned by this revelation, then talks in a more lively way than ever before. The doctor begins to feel a little warmer towards a patient he has always rather disliked.

In both these cases there has been a definite change in the doctor's attitude towards the patient. Ralph's doctor moves from a weary scepticism through a phase of exaggerated therapeutic optimism (about the drinking) to a mood of kindness towards the patient and a gentle concern about his terrors and his loneliness as his life moves towards its close. Stuart's doctor, in my second example, starts off feeling irritated, then becomes quite angry, even aggressive. Having got that into the open, he then seems to reach a better understanding of his own feelings about the patient. He relaxes the 'back pedal brake' and work is permitted to proceed more freely.

Another doctor presented a patient called Alison, whom he described unflatteringly as 'sort of untidy with stringy hair and a bit of a mess' in Chapter 2. Ten minutes into the interview he is thinking: 'Oh my God, one miserable girl who can't do a damn thing for anybody.' Alison bridles at the word 'useless' and lets him know that she is not only a competent housewife, but good at her job as well. The doctor becomes more involved and they are able to have an interesting exchange about dependency and how it makes her feel uncomfortable. There is uncertainty about whether she wants any more of this sort of attention, but something useful seems to have come out of 'a rather messy interview'. A somewhat tedious patient has become someone interesting and thought-provoking enough to bring to the group.

In a number of other cases the doctor's attitude seems to have shifted as a result of a surprise remark by the patient: some statement or expression of feeling which doesn't fit into the doctor's previous picture. Edna (in Chapter 2) shows herself capable of humour when the dishes crash down and thereafter becomes a more welcome guest in the surgery. Sarah's doctor in Chapter 8 was 'coasting along, thinking with relief that it would be a quick interview', when she told him that her adopted daughter was expecting a baby and then shocked him by being angry about it. Hannah's doctor (in Chapter 6) suddenly realizes that she is deaf and her deafness seems to throw into focus all her painful feelings about being lonely, old, and starved of affection. Fortunately, in each of these cases the doctors quickly recovered from their initial shock and were able to develop a greater concern and compassion for their patients.

Another shock occurs for the doctor in Chapter 4 when he describes a pair of sisters who are 'superficially similar', but one is married while the other is known to be single and to have a spinal deformity. When the second sister comes to the doctor he is given the wrong set of notes but manages to identify the lady correctly ('Oh dear, you're not Jean, are you?'). The patient replies: 'No, I'm Mary, the one who lives alone.' This sad little sentence has the effect of suddenly illuminating someone who had previously been in the shadows. The doctor feels a pang of sorrow for her which he will not forget. There seems little doubt that whenever he sees this patient in future the doctor will say to himself: 'Ah yes, Mary – the one that lives alone.' The one that lives alone has successfully claimed a belated recognition of her loneliness – and her uniqueness.

In another case, described in Chapter 8, the doctor surprises himself by informing a young mother with a sort of ex cathedra infallibility that her migraine attacks will never happen when she is alone with her children. This young woman has always appeared to her doctor as 'a jolly sort of athletic person . . . who hides a lot of anxieties under a hard shell.' He describes his bland reassurance as a crazy remark, as he can't possibly know whether she will have a migraine or not. Nevertheless the remark has a considerable result because the patient seems to soften a little and admits for the first time that she feels vulnerable and insecure when her husband is away. Initially the doctor felt that a new era was beginning in which Peggy would talk more freely about her anxieties. In the event this never happened, but in the course of the next year there were thirteen 'brief encounters' in which doctor and patient discussed her children's minor illnesses. The doctor reported that he now felt that he was an important person for her – someone she relied on to take care of her; 'to reassure her that everything will be alright'. Again we can't really know whether this is indeed the way she feels about him; but we have enough evidence to be confident that he will never again think of her as simply a bright, brittle, 'hockey stick' girl.

A dramatic change in the doctor's view of the patient is reported in Chapter 7. The patient, Vivienne, is introduced as a sort of caricature: she has 'a zombie-like appearance and manner – a combination of drugged behaviour and weird eye make-up'. She seems to be a hopeless addict whose life is dominated by 'booze, fags, and pills'. More in hope than expectation, the doctor suggests that she might try to cut down the pills and keep a record of the ones she takes together with any events which precipitate the need for them. Amazingly Vivienne responds by presenting her doctor with a detailed diary in which she records her daily struggles with her family, her symptoms, and her feelings. She reveals herself as a talented diarist and diarists can cast a particularly potent spell over their readers. This diary does not fail to make a powerful impression on the doctor who is, after all, its inspiration and its dedicatee. She now sees her patient, the erstwhile 'zombie', as someone capable of writing about her experiences in a vivid, expressive style which is eloquent and moving. In Vivienne's case, perhaps exceptionally, there is good evidence that the diary had had a therapeutic effect on its author: she has given up most of her drugs and is addressing her life with a new determination. But whatever else happens to Vivienne she will always be 'the woman who sent me that diary' as far as her doctor is concerned.

In all the cases I have quoted there seems to be genuine evidence of a change for the better in the doctor's attitude to the patient concerned. We still do not know really how the patients have fared. Is it possible to demonstrate a positive benefit for the patient as a result of the improvement in his doctor's condition? I think the most we can reasonably claim is that the doctor is likely to be more effective after his change of attitude, at least as long as it lasts. The changes we have seen have all been in the direction of a greater willingness to tolerate and accept the patient whether or not he responds to any conventional treatment (such as cures for alcoholism or depression) which may be on offer. The doctor is more willing 'to be a doctor for someone', without flailing around desperately 'trying to do something'.

In order to be a doctor for someone it is not sufficient just to have your name on their medical card. You have to be willing to sit still and soak up a lot of frustration, distress, and hopelessness. You have to be emotionally responsive while keeping your personal life unentangled with that of the patient. You also need to be around for a long enough period of time – anything from a few weeks to a lifetime. You still have to take a detailed interest in minor illnesses and respond reliably to major ones. And if, just occasionally, you can make an observation which is illuminating and share it with your patient – so much the better.

Leonard Woolf, after reflecting on what seemed to him to be a lack of solid achievements in his life, entitled the last volume of his autobiography *The Journey Not The Arrival Matters*. The metaphor of life as a journey has cropped up more than once already in these pages and I feel I may be excused for using it once again. Marie Campkin has described a patient who began with a request for a passport and then embarked on a journey so rapid and headlong that the doctor felt left behind. Oliver Samuel and Cyril Gill have portrayed the doctor as the careful helmsman giving 'A touch on the tiller' and trimming the sails. He can also be regarded as a useful person to have as a fellow traveller; able when necessary to help with the navigation or repair the engine, but mostly there to share the experience and help to reflect on it. He doesn't know, any more than the patient, how or where the journey will end; he is also on a journey of his own.

11
Research, changes, and development in Balint Groups[1]
Enid Balint

The aim of Balint groups has changed very little, if at all, over the last twenty years. Changes, however, have occurred in the techniques which the general practitioners study in the groups. It may be more of a surprise to find how little our thinking has changed than the way in which it has changed. I do not think this is due to our inflexibility.

What is general practice like? Andrew Elder describes it in Chapter 6 as a world where:

'the doctor is frequently in the dark, getting glimpses of his patients from time to time, being careful not to find out too much, being content to find out the right distance for the patient and for himself; sometimes taking the initiative, and at other times needing to be more restrained.' (p. 54)

If a doctor thinks that this task is one that he would like to undertake and that it is not too far from his ideas about general practice, a Balint group should be able to provide the means by which he can learn to do so.

I am assuming, of course, that such a doctor would be well-trained and continue to be interested in traditional medicine all of his professional life, because without that none of our ideas have their place in medicine, or can be used reliably.

I will explain briefly how we started. In 1949 Michael Balint led a group of non-medical professional workers at The Tavistock Clinic – a mixed group I had started in 1948 with the aim of trying to understand and work with people with marital difficulties. We then decided to start working with general practitioners using the same techniques we had developed during the previous work.

Our method of work and our research method were stable and consisted of discussion in a structured setting, of a doctor's difficulties

[1]This chapter is based on a paper first presented in October 1984 at the 6th International Balint Conference in Montreux.

with a patient; one particular relationship at one particular time. The same leader, the same doctors, discussed patients together in the same place over a longish period. Verbatim transcripts were made of each meeting.

We found the use of the doctor's own notes distracting during the discussion itself, and we soon adopted a method based on the method of supervision used by Hungarian psychoanalysts. This was to encourage students to speak freely without notes, contradict themselves if necessary, have second thoughts, remember things they thought they had forgotten; so that a complete picture emerged in which the feelings of the doctor himself were evident alongside the facts he was reporting.

If you have never worked like this with a leader trained to observe in a particular way, who can tolerate the absence of a consistent story for a time, and use the muddle rather than try to discard it, this method may sound very strange and unscientific. It consists of amassing facts and the feelings about the facts at the same time. Our work is based on the idea that human beings, whether doctors or patients, unconsciously defend themselves against certain thoughts and ideas. They try to get things in order and this often involves leaving out facts and the feelings about them. The story seems clear and the doctor when reporting is unaware that it is incorrect. In our kind of discussion and reporting, such omissions and falsifications come to light without embarrassment.

A trained observer – possibly a psychoanalyst or someone who has worked with one for a long time – is needed to help piece the data together. Hunches, fantasies, and feelings should be expressed without embarrassment but not treated as sacred. The work of the group and of the doctor in charge of the patient is to see if what is said is true – to examine on what such fantasies and hunches are based – so that the doctor can, if appropriate, change his ideas about his patient. This is all done in a stable setting, and each doctor gets accustomed to looking at his and his colleagues' work, with the same strictness and freedom.

We still use the same method. But do we listen in the 1980s in a different way for different things? Have we changed? We are, perhaps, even less anxious to make a coherent story, to make 'sense' early on in our work. We still make a working diagnosis, but we are now more observant of changes, however minute, which take place in the doctor–patient relationship – in the doctor's feelings about his patients and in the patients' complaints – even changes which take place during one consultation. We are particularly careful not to fit new observations into old patterns where they are inappropriate.

Early in our work we sometimes spoke about our ability to train general practitioners to do some form of psychotherapy and we blamed unsuccessful results on the fact that our doctors did not have much experience in this field. It was assumed then that had the 'psychotherapy' been better the patient would have been cured. The most common basis of any form of psychotherapy, it was said at the time, is an understanding of the patient's real problems. It was, therefore, thought that had these been understood the patient would have been helped. By 'real problems' was meant the underlying cause of the patient's illness. I now often think it is unnecessary and can be unhelpful at any given time to try to discover what a patient thinks is the cause of his present symptom or unhappiness. In general practice work the patient's feelings in the present, and the changes in them, seem more important and more reliable.

All our work is based on one human being – a professional, understanding not only intellectually but in other ways as well; medically, based on traditional medical teaching, and by identification. Intellectual understanding alone is not enough. To understand, one must listen to what one does not understand, watch, and notice the human being one is talking to and one's self at the same time; noticing and watching changes in one's ways of reacting to the other person. Identification depends more on a willingness, or even a desire to understand, than an ability to sympathize. However, once an observer has identified himself with someone or something, he will find it difficult to feel objectively about that person or thing again. So he must first identify and then he must withdraw from that identification and become an objective professional observer again. The identification must have a biphasic structure. In addition, a doctor must be able to respond correctly, without too much delay.

Scientists in other fields describe how difficult, or even impossible, it is to observe anything without influencing the object observed. No two observers will see exactly the same thing. The value of Balint groups is to facilitate observations.

I will describe a case.

It is a follow-up of a woman patient who had been seen and reported on almost a year before, soon after her first child was born: the baby, a girl, was suffering from a severe cough. The doctor had the cough 'investigated' but it continued. The patient continued to come to see the doctor complaining that she could not stand being kept awake at night any more. She must get back to work because she was no good at being a mother anyway, and she wanted to carry on with her career. Her husband was no help, either. The group had discussed this case the year before and had thought the patient was a rather overdominant, masculine woman (although there was no real evidence of her being masculine, other than her not being able to cope with her first child and wanting to go back to work). The working diagnosis was of a dominant woman with a weak husband who was presenting her child with a cough and who bullied her doctor. At the follow-up, however, the question of whether the woman was dominant came under review. Could it be taken for granted on the grounds that the doctor fitted in with her requests for frequent examinations of the child and anyway, the group asked this time, was this diagnosis of any help to the doctor or the patient? Most of the group were doubtful, but did not know where to turn, and then slowly began to look at the interview itself which the doctor was asked to report in greater detail. The doctor then told us that he thought the patient was very lonely. She had moved quite far from her home when she got married two years before, and the picture of the dominant, unattractive woman disappeared and we seemed to have somebody else as a patient. The doctor began to feel more at ease when he talked about her and said how lonely it must be for her. How awful it was for her to have a child and to have no one to share it with. He got in touch with feelings in himself and identified with the patient.

But there had been no biphasic structure in his identification with the patient, so he was not able to help her, only feel sorry for her. After the discussion in the group he could see how to help. The patient was then able to feel less alone with her husband, less lonely, and to let her husband share more.

I will give another case to illustrate this point.

A doctor reported on the case of an old patient of his, one he had known for several years, who, at the age of 36, was dying of cancer. She had had all the possible treatments and was now so distressed and so unwilling to go back into hospital that her general practitioner had advised that she be left at home until she died. The hospital had agreed to this. The doctor, however, then found it was very difficult for him to visit his patient and reported this case to the seminar because of his difficulty in visiting his dying patient. The seminar was very subdued and made all sorts of excuses for the doctor. They could well understand how, because he could do nothing for her, he could not bring himself to visit her: that he was very busy, and so on, and so on. The case was discussed for quite a long time before someone said he was sure the doctor wanted to visit the patient but was so identified with her he could not face it. The doctor agreed: yes, he wanted to go but he couldn't face the way she looked, although when he saw her he did not mind at all. In fact when he got into her bedroom he was very pleased to sit on her bed and hold her hand, which she put out towards him when he entered the room. He began to see her as a separate person whom he could be with; relate to. This doctor needed to realize that the patient was a separate person, and one who did not expect anything of him he could not give; a person who was glad to have somebody with her who could accept the fact that she was dying, and that she did not look too frightening. There was no need for him to say anything special. We will come back to this.

When did we begin to observe the changes in our focus of interest, changes in the techniques we were trying to devise for general practitioners? It is difficult to say, but a new appraisal started in January 1966, when a research team consisting of ten general practitioners and two, sometimes three, psychoanalytic leaders met at University College Hospital under the leadership of Michael Balint and myself. The group ended in 1971, a year after Michael Balint died. A book, *Six Minutes for the Patient*, based on the research in the group, was published in 1973.

The new techniques that we were aiming at had to be based on a reliable understanding of the patient's individuality and particularly of the developing relationship between the patient and the doctor, that is to say on processes rather than states. The time needed for these techniques had to be compatible with the routine ten minutes or so that the average patient gets in a medical practice. We encountered severe difficulties in this group; the principal one was caused perhaps by the realization that their old well-proven methods had to be given up, or at any rate considerably modified. This was partly because of the new conditions and partly because we were not sure whether the results in the long run gave the doctor, and therefore the patient, sufficient satisfaction. In the old method which we were giving up, the doctor had responsibility for understanding not only what the patient tried to convey to him, but why the patient had become the way he was. Although he was as interested as we still were, to recognize omissions and distortions in the patient's story, his aim then was to solve something, which is, after all, the traditional role of the doctor. But in the new technique the therapist's role was to tune in to the patient and to see what it was like both for himself and for the patient and what changes occurred and how varied and inconsistent his feelings and the stories that he got were. The need here to identify and then withdraw from the identification is paramount. The technique which arose out of these ideas was called the 'flash' and consisted of a moment of mutual understanding between a doctor and his patient which was *communicated by the doctor to his patient*. It was not an understanding about the patient's past about which the doctor was very likely completely aware, but was usually about something in the patient's current life and which was reflected in the relationship with the doctor for a brief time. These episodes were very hard to follow up reliably, but when they have been followed up changes do seem to persist in the doctor's feelings about the patient, but we have not been able to observe reliably in what way the patient responded to them. It appeared that they were sometimes brushed aside: not referred to again.

In the research reported in this book and in research being undertaken at the present time the focus is on a technique similar, in some ways, to the *flash* technique: but different in important ways. We are now more concerned with making observations about changes that take place in a doctor's feelings about his patient and a patient's feelings about his doctor; changes which *are not communicated at the time by the doctor to the patient.* This is crucial.

In the *flash* technique, when a flash occurred the doctor communicated his thoughts and feelings to the patient. Nowadays we prefer to wait and see what happens to a patient when a doctor's feelings change – sometimes suddenly – about him.

Here is another case, that of Hannah (see Chapter 6).

A woman in her late 60s, married to a man eight years younger than the patient. This woman had come complaining of depression for many years, for which she had been given pills and which she had said had always helped her. The doctor had changed the medication from time to time and each time the patient seemed satisfied, although she came back again with the same symptom. One day, however, the patient came as usual – or so it seemed – and the doctor found himself asking her whether there was something that was particularly wrong. The patient said her husband had a mistress, but this kind of thing had happened so often before she did not think it had any particular significance, and she spoke in a way that did not make the doctor feel that she was particularly troubled by it. But at that time the doctor found himself seeing the patient as an old woman with a deaf-aid (which he himself had given her some years before); a woman who felt that her life was over with her husband who would never want her any more; that there could be no more sexual relationship between them; and that she was finished. Actually, it was the doctor who felt all of this and who reported these feelings at some length to the group. We did not know what the patient felt. In this interview the doctor had not said anything about this to his patient, but he was shocked. He did not suppose that the patient was aware of any of this at the time, but the group felt that probably the patient had felt old and useless many times and that it was the doctor who had only just picked it up. Perhaps the patient felt better because of this. The patient returned in three weeks' time and said that she was depressed, but for the first time said that the pills were no good and that there was no point in her having any more. She had come because she was going on holiday with her husband and she wanted to talk to the doctor first about it, but she did not want to use pills. The patient said she was terrified that she was going to spoil the holiday. Her husband had planned it after giving up his relationship with his girlfriend and this made the patient particularly anxious that she should not spoil it; that the better relationship which seemed to be growing between her and her husband should not be spoiled by her being so awful and depressed and useless.

In this interview the patient showed something which could have been caused by the doctor's feelings in the interview before, when he had felt despair for her and fear for her future but had said nothing. We could say that the patient had 'unloaded' her feelings into the doctor and in consequence she had become partially free of them and was able (instead of being passive about them) to become active as if free for the time being and not passively having to accept her fate. If this was so, this was a major change. The idea is that what the doctor 'took in' during that interview had afterwards enabled the patient to be free enough to take the initiative at the next interview (by not accepting the pills as usual); and also to behave differently, more actively, less like a victim with her husband in the meantime. The doctor, having had insight into the patient's ideas about herself (not about what she was like, but what she felt she was like), enabled her to come alive and to rid herself, temporarily at any rate, of her heavy, passive depression. The doctor had, so to speak, taken in what the patient projected into him and had held onto it for a time; had not immediately handed it back to the patient in the form of an interpretation. At the next interview, however, when she came saying she did not want the pills but did not want to be depressed, he was able to respond appropriately, having by that time got rid of the patient's depression. He did not, of course, say 'you are an old, deaf woman and there is no hope for you', but spoke about the holiday and the processes that were going on inside the patient, at that time.

There have been other cases, as I have already shown in this chapter, which confirm our ideas about this particular kind of tuning in. One could talk about it in terms of the doctor being willing to accept and to hold on to feelings given him by a patient during a consultation, and examining these feelings before withdrawing from them, or isolating himself from them. We then have to examine the effect this has on the patient; namely when the doctor does not interpret but holds on to feelings which a patient has aroused in him, and with which, for a short time, he totally identifies but which he is able to distance himself from later. He knows what it is like to be the patient but also is able to see that that is not all the patient has inside him. The doctor must become aware of the feelings the patient has, and be ready to hear what the patient says at the next consultation as well. The patient can then become the active one and is not deflated by accepting something about herself passively; or, if that is too threatening, by having to fail to take it seriously at all. The patient can change once the doctor knows what it is like to feel the way she does. She can then tune in to other parts of herself. But she cannot change, sometimes, by being told that she should change, or being told what she is like. She is given the freedom to change in this way.

This brings me back to another reason why we run our groups the way we do. It is so that the doctors in the groups can be active, not passively receptive, either of their own feelings or to what the leader says. They can talk freely about their patients and their feelings about them, at one particular moment, in one particular session, bearing in mind that this is almost certain to change. In so doing they can get in touch with feelings in themselves about which they have been unaware and which may enable them in due course to understand something about their patients which they would not have been able to do, had they been out of touch with their own feelings and the seriousness of them.

To take the responsibility for their own feelings and thoughts, to realize how hard it is to observe them reliably, how easy it is to miss what other people say: these are some of the things that doctors in Balint groups get to know about. Balint groups allow such processes to occur, allow doctors to realize how hard it is to observe, particularly when the observations are not stable. In this work activity of a special kind is released in the doctors, a kind of psychic activity. Liveliness: not passive acceptance. Observations: not instructions.

12
My troubled patients: Do I really help them?

John Salinsky

It is now about eleven years since I joined my first Balint group. My intention at that time was to learn a technique of psychotherapy which I could apply to some troubled patients who were also troubling me. Some of them were people with persistent physical symptoms for which there were no organic explanations and apparently no cure. Others told me quite frankly that they were troubled by a lack of emotional satisfaction which they wanted me to put right – preferably with a simple course of tablets, but if this was not possible, by any other means that I could recommend.

After the first few weeks of the group's existence I became discontented. I seemed to be discovering, like my unfortunate patients, that no simple formula was on offer. At first I protested, again rather like my patients, that the group leaders must surely know the *answers*. Why did they not simply reveal their knowledge to their disciples so that we could apply it to the satisfaction of all concerned? Eventually I was persuaded (almost) that the leaders were also groping in semi-darkness; trying as best they could to make sense of the patients' communications and our reactions to them. I settled down to discussing the cases and presenting some of my own. Gradually I began to learn more about the things that go on in the course of a doctor–patient relationship. I found that these dialogues between doctor and patient were themselves of great interest and richness – even if I never entirely understood what they were about. The fact that one couldn't often solve the patient's problems seemed to matter less; the people became more interesting than the 'diseases' and my daily work with difficult patients began to make a new kind of sense. Since those early days I have been in a number of other groups and have graduated to leading groups for trainee general practitioners. Many of the other doctors I talk to are also Balint graduates and we all seem to feel enjoyment from our work. But sometimes, amid this rather congenial medical satisfaction, I find myself wondering whether the patients have somehow got lost.

I don't seem to have found a way of asking them whether they feel any better, or indeed less troubled, for having had the benefit of a general practitioner with a training in understanding the doctor–patient relationship. What, for example, has happened to all those patients whom I presented to that original group in the mid-70s? I resolved to try and find out.

When I looked through my transcripts and other records I discovered that I had presented a total of nine patients in the course of four years. Most of these had also been the subject of follow-up reports and hence further discussion. Unfortunately five out of the nine have subsequently left the district. I propose to examine three of the remaining four, excluding the fourth because she has already been described in a previous paper. I shall replace her with a man (the other three are all women). He is someone whom I met after the group had dissolved and would surely have been presented if I'd had the opportunity. Furthermore, my unconscious has recommended him for inclusion in a very determined way. I can make no other excuse for such an outrageous betrayal of my resolution to be totally objective and will have to leave the reader to judge whether I did rightly. At any rate all four were deeply troubled patients when I met them between seven and twelve years ago. Did I really help them?

INGRID

Ingrid was 37 when I first met her. She had been born in Denmark and had lived in England since her late teens. Her marriage to an Englishman had ended in divorce a year before we met and she had one 7 year-old daughter. At first she wanted 'treatment' to get rid of some disagreeable physical sensations which included blushing, sweating, and palpitations which occurred whenever she was nervous and particularly when she was talking to someone she wanted to impress. Before long we were talking about her distress that she had nobody to love her. She seemed unable to find a replacement for her allegedly 'cold and selfish' husband. Ingrid was one of my earliest cases and I was eager to get straight to the heart of the doctor–patient relationship. Rather clumsily I asked her how she felt about me and was disconcerted when she said she often felt like putting her arms around me! The same evening she telephoned me at home and invited me to go to a concert with her. I declined rather stiffly and said that we must confine our relationship to the professional one in the surgery. When I reported these exchanges to the group, they became quite excited and interrogated me closely about what had made me ask such a stupid question in the first place. My answers failed to satisfy them. They seemed to feel that Ingrid was a hopeless, pathetic creature who inspired revulsion rather than pity or concern. My optimism about the prognosis was regarded as totally unrealistic and I returned from the group feeling bruised.

Nevertheless, I went on seeing Ingrid at fortnightly intervals for several years. She told me about a succession of sad love affairs in which her romantic feelings were either spurned or cynically exploited. The two longest affairs were with a married man who was clearly not going to leave his wife, and with a manipulative hemiplegic man who seemed to enjoy making Ingrid feel totally dependent on him. She had other more promising friendships, but frequently alienated people by her tendency to be prickly and suspicious when asked about her personal life. In the course of our conversations I tried to point out the way in which she set emotional traps for herself and predictably fell into them. 'How can I change, then? What must I do?', she would demand, tearfully and indignantly. I knew what needed changing, but of course I didn't know how. After a couple of years of fortnightly half-hour sessions at the end of surgery, I told her that I didn't think I could solve her problems. Would she like to be referred for psychotherapy? No, she didn't want anyone but me. I reduced the frequency of her sessions to once a month and later, with her agreement, to once in three months until the regular appointments petered out. In the last few years she has turned up spontaneously about three times a year and I have usually been able to find about half an hour for her. Nine years on, she is still alone, apart from her daughter, now taking A-levels. She has a steady job as a teacher in a girls' school – which she says she hates. She has never invited me out again, but she did for a while have a social relationship with my wife whom she met at a literary club. And we were both invited to meet Ingrid's fiancé – a few weeks before she angrily returned his ring. About six months ago she came for one of her sporadic consultations and said that she still had nobody to love her and that her life was empty. I said I felt sorry that in our eleven years as doctor and patient I had been of so little help. 'Without you to talk to,' she responded, with some emotion, 'I don't know how I would have survived. I would have gone crazy.'

If I did help Ingrid, how did I manage it? Clearly not by finding out what was 'really' wrong with her. Not by making pseudoanalytical interpretations (although I made plenty of those in the early days). I suppose I helped her because I stayed with her and I was able to do that because I was interested in her and moved by her feelings. My interest, my concern for her, and my willingness to share her feelings must, I think, have to do with a feeling of identification which I had with her. I shall return to this idea a little later on.

CORA

Cora was a lady of 52, unmarried, and living with her younger sister in a large old house which had belonged to their parents. When she first appeared in my surgery I was struck by the way her rather pointed features were twisted into a grimace of distress. 'My doctor won't have me any more,' she said, 'because I've been in too many hospitals. And I make too much noise when I cry.' It emerged that the hospitals were psychiatric establishments and her diagnosis according to her records had progressed from 'hysterical personality' to 'paranoid schizophrenia' over the course of ten years. That initial encounter ended with her crying (noisily, but not for long), and asking if she could come again in a fortnight. She came regularly and I soon got to know her better. I heard about her tiring, tedious job as a cleaner in a large canteen and her demented mother who had to be visited regularly in a geriatric ward on the other side of London. After a few months she suddenly became quite psychotic with delusions about soldiers landing by parachute in her back garden. Her sister was unable to cope with her and so I had her admitted to the local institution. A few days later something prompted me to visit her there. This is not something I normally do as the hospital is half an hour's drive away and not all that easy to find. Eventually I located the right ward and entered cautiously. Cora recognized me at once and dissolved into noisy tears. She grasped both my hands in her claw-like fingers and with her face twisting up into the now familiar spasm of grief she sobbed: 'Take me home. I don't like it here.'

I had a few words with the staff who were grateful for my interest and she was discharged home the next day. Shortly afterwards she was joined in the surgery by her sister who must have felt left out of our sessions. Now they always come together. Every other Wednesday afternoon I find them sitting side by side in my waiting room, handbags clutched tightly on their knees, waiting for their appointment. 'How are you today?' I ask. 'Not very good, doctor,' they answer in chorus. Then Cora says: 'Will I have to go back into hospital?'

She has not been back for eight years, thanks partly to depot phenothiazines, but thanks also, I would suggest, to those fortnightly conversations, mostly less than ten minutes in length. How, I wonder, was I able to develop a lasting relationship with someone so grotesquely miserable? The group, to whom I presented Cora, were quick to seize on the mental hospital visit as the crucial event which engaged my sympathy. But when I think about it now I am reminded immediately of an episode in my own childhood. At the age of three or four I had also been 'sent away' – to a children's home while my mother was ill. While I was there, suffering acutely from separation pains, I developed a severe gastroenteritis and was brought back, more dead than alive, by my guilt-ridden parents. Or so the family legend relates. At any rate the dim memories of this episode are still enough to make me slightly queasy when I think about it and I feel fairly certain that I was able to share with Cora an intense dread of being 'sent away' and a corresponding yearning to be 'taken home'.

MRS STERN

When I first met them in 1975 the Sterns were a couple of central European origin in their 60s and without children. Mr Stern had ischaemic heart disease and had recently had a stroke which had almost totally deprived him of speech. Nevertheless one could see that he had a warm friendly personality and he did his best to communicate in spite of his cruel disability. After my first visit we all seemed to be getting on well and Mrs Stern asked if they could become my 'private' patients. I told them that I had no private patients and was indeed opposed to private practice, being a loyal supporter of the National Health Service and the Labour Party which had created it. Mrs Stern said that they too believed in the NHS and had always voted Labour. Nevertheless she felt that general practitioners were too busy and under too much pressure to be able to provide the kind of attention her husband needed. If I was willing to give them a little extra time and trouble, she would see that I was properly rewarded. Naturally I refused any *ex gratia* payments.

I determined to show Mrs Stern that I could give her husband a first rate service entirely within the scope and rules of the National Health Service. Unfortunately they lived very much on the fringe of the practice territory and every visit meant a long and tedious drive, sometimes in heavy traffic. There were many requests for emergency visits, often without, at least in my view, any good reason except Mrs Stern's anxiety about her husband. More than once I became quite angry with her for calling me out unnecessarily. She seemed to have a special knack of saying things which made me feel irritated. And she seemed to be successfully making her point that it was impossible to be a 'good' doctor without being paid extra for special favours. Then on one of these annoying 'false alarm' visits Mr Stern turned out to be quite ill with left ventricular failure. When I suggested admission to hospital, he shook his head vehemently and let me know that he would like me to look after him at home. He was so nice that I agreed without hesitation. There followed a few weeks of frequent visiting and intensive treatment, not without a few more acerbic exchanges with Mrs Stern. Fortunately Mr Stern recovered some of his strength and expressed his appreciation warmly. Mrs Stern thanked me as well, but as usual she managed to offend me in the same sentence. 'You are a good doctor,' she said, 'but you have no psychology.' What a deplorable thing to say to a 'Balint' doctor! I crept away, mortified and indignant.

Eventually Mr Stern's heart succumbed after a long struggle. Mrs Stern had time to consider her own health. She had suffered from mild angina for several years but had suppressed her own symptoms for fear of alarming her husband. Now she wanted to know why I had not 'done something about it years ago'. She also wanted prescriptions for various vitamins to relieve her tiredness. When I protested that they were useless she said, 'No, that can't be true. All my friends get them from their doctors. Some of them are older than me and yet they can do more than I can. They cannot understand why you are so unwilling to help me.'

This was too much. I pointed out to her all the help I had given her over the years and reproached her for her ingratitude.

She paused for a moment and then said, 'You have never liked me, have you? I have never understood why. You have never wanted to know anything about me as a person. You think I am just a miserable whining old woman, but I can tell you there is more to me than that, a lot more. For instance I am a trained violinist and still give lessons. I am very fond of art and antiques which my husband and I used to collect. All these things we could have talked about if you had wanted. I would like to ask you to come and have tea with me, not as a doctor but just as an ordinary person, so I can show you what I am really like.'

The following week I went round for tea as an ordinary person. I could see that she was very pleased that I had accepted. She said, 'My friends all told me you wouldn't come, but I knew that you would. In spite of everything, we have a bond between us, you and I. Together we kept my husband alive for a few more years. He liked you very much and I think that you liked him also.' I confirmed that this was true. She went on talking about him and herself and me for about an hour, but I never really discovered why I had not got to know her 'as a person'.

She had decided that I was not really interested in the human side of medicine and it seemed useless to protest that there were lots of other patients whom I felt that I knew very well as 'people'. Why didn't it happen with Mrs Stern? Not because we had nothing in common. Anybody who could engage my feelings as strongly as she did must be very close to me in some obscure way. Perhaps she reminds me of a part of myself which I would prefer not to acknowledge. I will move hurriedly on to my last patient about whom I feel much more comfortable (but I promise to return to Mrs Stern before I close).

MR BOWMAN

The original patient was Mrs Bowman, a gentle fair-haired lady who developed cardiac failure in her early 70s and teetered on the brink of existence for several years. Her drug regime needed a good deal of fine tuning as she developed adverse reactions to some hypertensive agents and needed large doses of diuretics to prevent breathlessness.

To provide the necessary supervision I used to visit her regularly once a month. During each visit I would examine her heart and lungs, check her blood pressure, and write out a prescription for the next month's supply of drugs. As I was writing, Mr Bowman, her husband, would pour out two glasses of Guinness (one for me, one for himself) from a bottle carefully placed to warm up on the radiator. The three of us would then have a pleasant chat for a few minutes after which I would depart with an inner glow – owing something to the Guinness and a good deal to the warmth and cheerfulness of the Bowmans.

Unhappily Mrs Bowman's heart found the struggle increasingly difficult. She developed renal failure and had to be admitted to hospital where she died. The following week I went to see the bereft widower on the usual day at the usual time. This time he sat in her chair and told me about their fifty years of happy marriage. We had our glass of Guinness and toasted her memory. I thought that my professional task now was to do a bereavement job. Mr Bowman needed to be guided in an orderly manner through the various stages of grief (shock, anger, depression, acceptance, etc.) after which he would resume an active life as a socially reintegrated widower, supported by his family, and going to day centres, lunch clubs, etc. when he needed any outside stimulation.

Somehow it didn't quite work out like that. Although he was able to express his grief quite freely, Mr Bowman never progressed through any stages and never seemed to get his life together again. He remains a solitary and lonely figure, his life frozen at the moment when he lost his Dorothy. They seem to have lived a very self-contained life as a couple and scarcely needed anyone else. They had only one son who was married but had provided no grandchildren (a great pity because Mr Bowman likes talking to children and showing them conjuring tricks). Furthermore he and his daughter-in-law 'don't get on', so invitations are limited to once a year on Christmas Day. He has a home help and neighbours drop in to see if he needs anything; he gets his lunch at the pub sometimes, but mostly he is on his own. It is now five years since Mrs Bowman died and I am still visiting once a month –

and drinking my glass of Guinness. Sometimes we talk: about his wartime experiences, about his young days, about his health (I made him give up smoking for the sake of his bronchitis); and sometimes we talk about Dorothy. I must have got to know them both a few years after my own father died. I hadn't appreciated till then how devastating the loss of a beloved spouse can be; or how much love there can be between two ordinary people who have been together for a long time. I could feel Mr Bowman's loneliness and loss of Dorothy very acutely and I think he must be aware of this because sometimes we don't talk at all; we just sit there looking at each other and sipping our Guinness. Sometimes his face lights up in a wonderful smile after one of these silences. Sometimes his sadness brings tears to my eyes. The experience is a little painful but not something I want to run away from. My identification with him is somehow acceptable and the sharing of feelings is harmonious.

Our relationship is very different from the one I have with Mrs Stern and yet the two stories are superficially very similar. In each case I treated a patient with cardiac failure with the help of the spouse and was then needed to support the widowed partner. Both survivors were troubled patients, yet it seems that I could help only one of them. Perhaps at this point I should look again at all four cases. Did I help them and if so what did I do that was helpful? Did I solve any of their problems? I don't think so. Did I find out what was 'really' wrong with them and explain it to them so that they could dispense with their symptoms? No, that didn't happen either. I tried explaining things to Ingrid for quite a long time but it didn't make any difference. What did happen was that I found her interesting, responded to her feelings and was able to let her pour them out in the knowledge that they would be safely contained and treated with consideration. As I have already suggested, I think I was able to do this because of a strong sense of identification which I had with her. It was as though I could accept her feelings because they seemed to be part of me anyway. This is not to say that I was also suffering from unrequited love, but somewhere in my heart I remembered what it felt like – and I didn't find it too unbearable to experience.

In the same way with Cora I was able to accommodate some of her noisy crying without flinching and her distress about being exiled in an institution I recognized with particular poignancy. I have already described how Mr Bowman's widowhood seems to be part of me because of my feelings about my own parents being separated by death. The question which remains to be answered is why I was unable to help Mrs Stern if, as I believe, there was a strong identification with her also. As I think about this, I am reminded of Jung's concept of the Shadow which he described as personifying 'everything that the subject refuses to acknowledge about himself and yet is always thrusting itself upon him directly or indirectly'. (Collected Works, Vol. 9: 284) Could it have been that Mrs Stern represented or reminded me of part of my unacceptable 'Shadow' self? I can see that the effect she had on me was often to make me feel callous and uncaring. The only way I could escape from the associated guilt feelings seemed to be to obey her every wish like a little servant – which I found humiliating. It occurs to me that she herself may have had uncomfortable feelings like this herself, perhaps in relation to the way life (and the Nazis) had treated her, and that she was seeking relief by giving them to me to hold for her. If so, they were feelings that I did not understand and was by no means willing to recognize as having anything to do with me. I could accept and share Ingrid's yearning to be loved and Cora's dread of being sent away; I could even participate in Mr Bowman's widowhood. But Mrs Stern's feeling of guilt and humiliation (if that's what they were) were too much for me. Perhaps if I had understood them better I would have been able to appreciate the postive regard which she had for me as well.

My conclusion at the end of this reappraisal is that my ability to help my troubled patients is related – in a complex way – to my capacity to accept a share in their painful feelings. This may happen more readily if the patient is someone whose difficulties remind me of part of myself. But if the shared feelings are too painful; if they call attention to part of myself which I am not ready to acknowledge; or if I am pressed to take too heavy a share – then I push the feelings away and no helpful work can be done. I have described all this in relation to myself but I feel fairly confident that I am not 'a special case' and that these processes go on in just the same way with other doctors and other patients. Nor is it surprising that the patients we select (or our unconscious selects) for presentation at a Balint group are those who remind us of aspects of ourselves. This is particularly obvious to a group leader who often finds that members of his group will present different examples of 'the same case' one after another, as if they are trying to work through a persisting problem of their own. (Come to think of it, that is exactly what I have been doing myself in the course of this paper!) The group leader will also notice that sometimes the presenting doctor is so closely enmeshed with the patient that he seems hardly able to keep his own identity separate. In other cases the doctor is violently repelled as if he and the patient were like magnetic poles, unable to get close. The professional and personal skills which we all need constantly to improve are those of sharing our patients' feelings sufficiently to be able to help them without also merging with them completely. To refine these skills we need quietly to reflect from time to time on our own troubled feelings.

Appendix:
What happened to the patients?

Fact or fiction?

ALISON
The doctor's final report was that she had attended once more (with a sick child). Then, four months later, she came to ask if she and her family could remain as patients even though they were moving to a better house in another district. The doctor explained that this was not possible and she thanked him warmly for looking after them.

EDNA
Edna is now eighty. The frequency of her visiting has dropped considerably; in 1983 she attended the surgery three times, in the previous five years she attended between ten and seventeen times a year. This summer she has attended more frequently following a fall which resulted in bruising of her left knee and shoulder. She tore her supra-spinatus muscle, and this required a hydrocortisone injection, but this has now settled rather to my surprise, and we seem to have rather a comfortable relationship. Her heavy envelope no longer represents a burden.

MICHAEL
For a long time I had no personal contact with him, though I had to provide a medical report when he lost his job through being asked to work under conditions impossible for him − alone in a building at night. I have seen him a couple of times since. He is polite and friendly and says his travel problems are better, but he hasn't managed to get another job. I felt he was 'in control' of the consultation and was not looking for anything beyond this superficial level.

Search or serendipity?

MRS ISAACS
We established a relationship which enabled me to remember her and

chat about her family, but she soon lapsed into heart failure and slight dementia, for better or worse. Since then she has become more like the others in the home, but less aware of it.

LAURA

The immediate result of that first joint interview with Laura and her husband was that he really tried to be actively helpful. When they came next time it was obvious that they had been talking about their feelings more openly. They wanted to discuss with me what might happen if Laura became pregnant again. Would she become depressed and how could they prevent that happening? They also talked a good deal about how angry they both felt with both sets of their parents for being unhelpful and unconcerned. I thought that they were frustrated because they were unable to depend on their parents to help them and that they might want to depend on their doctor for a time instead. I said nothing but accepted that as my role and offered to see both of them regularly once a month for a time.

Two sessions later they came to tell me that Laura was pregnant and the whole situation had changed. She was much more confident outwardly and was coping well at work. She still had worries about how she would cope with two children. I took that to show her continuing need for support and I arranged to go on seeing them together, as well as arranging antenatal care. Soon we were talking about the way ruminating about babies had invaded her business time as Laura bloomed into pregnancy. She then had to go into hospital for a rest and suffered a set-back. Fears closed in around her and her husband came worried to tell me about it. I went to see her in the ward and spent an hour with her.

Fortunately she soon was home again and in due course was safely delivered of a second son. The baby was quickly established on the bottle ('so much easier if I have to go in to the office') and she adjusted quickly to being an efficient mother to her new baby and to coping with the tantrums of the older child. Soon she was back at the office for a couple of days each week, having a wonderful regular minder for the children. Clearly the dilemma of being pulled between the need to be a good enough mother and a dynamic business executive was still testing her.

Inexorably she became depressed and was offered time to talk through the problems and later was prescribed some antidepressant medication as well. Her husband did his best to help but had to be away from home on business all too often. Slowly over the next year the mood lifted and she now sees herself more as a mother who needs to escape to the office, than a full-time executive. Our regular sessions have stopped as have the prescriptions for drugs, but we still meet at the Well Baby clinic. She still has an occasional moan about the difficulty of maintaining a dual role and she has resumed half-time work in her profession. Last time we met she told me with a wry grimace that they were working out when the best time would be to start the next baby!

I feel I still have an important relationship with this couple, even though we no longer meet very often. I am a kind of background supporter, available to be conjured up for some extra help if they go through a bad patch, but not particularly needed just now.

MARY

The lady with the limp, who alerted the doctor by her remark 'I'm Mary, the one that lives alone.' She was ready to talk. A close friend had breast cancer, and she had just learnt that it was terminal. She has come four times since the reported interview, and the friend has now died. In her mourning she has also mourned her own lost opportunities. She says that it would be foolish to deny that her deformity has made life difficult, yet she would hate to say, 'Poor me, how could I possibly do any better?' We talk about many things, and she says the limp is not really so important, yet we always seem to come back to it. She feels that other people dislike her because she is either denying her problem rather stupidly, or displaying it, and feeling sorry for herself. I can easily identify these feelings in both of us. However, I seem to be trapped as a doctor, just as she is trapped by her deformity, and I cannot relate these feelings to other things in her life, which might give us another perspective. Her resentment makes us go round in circles rather annoyingly, and I hope for a breakthrough. We are at least slowly getting to know each other.

JANE

In a subsequent interview a few weeks later she told me that her father had been severely depressed after her mother's death in childbirth – she had been afraid that he would die too. She herself had had a 'nervous breakdown' a month after her marriage; there had been panic, nameless fears, and constant crying. She was very much afraid of this happening again. I continued to see her about twice a month and also referred her to a psychosexual specialist whom she saw once with her husband and several times on her own.

About a year after the reported interview she and her husband began to have intercourse successfully, although infrequently. I continued talking to her and supplying her with sleeping tablets about once a month, and about eight months later she became pregnant. Twin boys were successfuly delivered by Caesarian Section! The next few months were full of sleepless nights, endless baby feeding, and worry about their health (one of them had a heart murmur, fortunately innocent). When I last saw her, the twins were 5 months old, thriving well, and sleeping through the night. Jane looked happy and relaxed and was sleeping well herself – with the aid of one tablet.

The touch on the tiller

ROSE

Not seen again since the reported interview. This is in keeping with her occasional use of the doctor in moments of crisis.

SIMON AND GERALD

The homosexual partners. Fluctuating bouts of contact with both of them continue. Gerald is obsessed with death, and though he denies it, he really needs his arthritis and other non-lethal diseases, so that Simon and I have a valid context for looking after him. The dog, too, is getting old and weary, and carries some of the gloom superbly. Simon looks much younger than his age. His aches and pains are supposed to be due to over-exertion. However, he came to see me soon after his birthday and said he was depressed about Gerald and the dog, and yes, about being seventy too.

Conflict or collaboration?

MRS FRIEDMAN

Three-and-a-half years have elapsed since the reported interview. She and her husband have continued coming to see me about once a month. The husband pleaded with me to refer her to a hospital department where she could have the much desired hydrotherapy 'so that I can have a bit of peace'. I agreed and she seemed to enjoy the treatment, although she grumbled about the long ambulance journey and there was no lasting improvement in her symptoms. I allow her to grumble and do what I can for her symptoms, but there has been no further discussion about what sort of 'horrible person' she might be or why. Sometimes she is depressed, less often cheerfully defiant. Her one further flash of humour has been to award me the OBE for a successful venepuncture.

HILDA

She continued to attend every two months or so with her usual symptoms and occasional problems with her flat. One day she said she felt a very old lady – forgetting things and dropping things – but despite harassment from a new landlord, she 'won't move from the house until she goes for good'.

In 1984 she had a hospital admission for cardiac arrhythmia, and again in 1985 with a small infarct. She emerged, having lost some weight but undiminished in spirit, and continues as before.

LESLEY

She occasionally has a few pills for her back, but seems to be extremely self-sufficient. The baby has been seen a few times by various people in the practice, possibly because appointments were made at short notice, though she may prefer not to be involved with one particular doctor. When I have seen her it has been brief and matter of fact, with no reference to past events.

MARTHA

Martha found a lover, but unfortunately developed a pelvic inflammatory disease as a result. It seems he also drank heavily. She has been able to share these disasters with her doctor as they happened, one by one, and she has also been able to get rid of her unsatisfactory friend. She is worried about her son who has beaten up his young wife once or twice, and dreads history repeating itself. The doctor is relieved that she has not crept back into her tight little shell, but otherwise the outlook seems gloomy.

Moments of change

RALPH

During the next year he had three emergency hospital admissions for gastrointestinal bleeding, brought on by bouts of drinking. In between there were varying periods of abstinence – one lasted seven weeks, but ended abruptly when his flat was flooded in a freak rainstorm, and he went out at once and got drunk. He would come every two or three weeks to report progress, and it was always clear as he came in the door whether things were going well or badly, by his jaunty or defeated step. He stopped making protestations about 'never touching another drop' but would ask from time to time about his prognosis and agree solemnly when I said it rather depended on how he treated his fragile stomach and liver.

In the following year he had three more episodes of bleeding, culminating in an operation – oesophageal transection. From that time he had a period of abstinence for over a year before lapsing, and has had a few brief binges since. He sees me regularly every month for sleeping pills, and the relationship remains friendly but low-key. Sometimes he talks about his rather empty life or about past events. He makes no promises and both his and my expectations are modest. I have not offered him any kind of 'repeat prescription' arrangement because I feel his brief monthly visits are mutually reassuring; for me, about his continued well-being, and for him as evidence of my continued concern.

STUART

Stuart now works in a hospital CSSD (instrument sterilizing) department and continues to have many difficulties. Life never seems easy for him nor is my task as his doctor. Consultations now seem to occur in clusters quite close to each other and then ease off for a while. There was sometimes a run of consultations before a holiday or going away with a friend. The reported interviews do seem to have been a turning point. I have known him for quite a few years. This may be a relationship of some importance to him in what seems like a pretty restricted life. I still often find him exasperating but get less angry, and am happier with a longer-term and less ambitious perspective.

The reported interviews led on to a series of about five further longish interviews in which his constant dread of serious illness became more apparent, a morbid preoccupation. The hospital wasn't a place of safety for him as I had imagined, but rather a place of constant danger, in which he felt trapped. He becomes very anxious about new illnesses, and was worried about AIDS at one stage, feeling he could share this anxiety with no one. He seems to feel 'trapped' or 'stuck' all round, a feeling which was clearly reflected in how stuck I had felt with him at the beginning of the reports, and often have done since. In relation to work he feels unable to stay where he is and panicky, but unable to leave and move on. More recently, he has again taken steps to change jobs, and this time has actually applied for further training in computer work. He seems to need help from doctors but makes life difficult for them by not trusting them much.

He appears to have no close friends and has begun to rely again more on his parents, whom he frequently visits as they are becoming more frail. He talks about them occasionally and the serious illnesses they both have, but seems to get only confusing information about them from their doctors who don't seem to offer enough help.

On two occasions things have got particularly bad. At one point he developed sciatic pain from a nerve root compression and had a difficult time for about four months, ending up as an in-patient for traction and eventually a successful epidural block. There was much helpless anxiety during these months, many telephone calls, and muddle between different opinions and further consultations at either the hospital or with me at the surgery. On one occasion these included a fearful image of himself as a 'life-long invalid'.

After this episode resolved there were no consultations for about five months, and then a deepening depression seemed to occur, with weight loss and increasing sleeplessness. He was on the point of packing up and going home to live with his parents. A neighbour was becoming intolerable, driving him mad with music from next door, and at work he had to hide with unpredictable bouts of crying. He seemed ill and I saw him often as well as prescribing anti-depressants. He seemed to respond well and after a few weeks was better. During these consultations he realized he found talking helpful for the first time. Over the next few months we thought about him joining a psycho-therapy group. He considered it, saw the group leader, panicked a few times, considered it again, and eventually started in the group, which he has now been attending for over a year. I saw him occasionally in the early days of this starting but not now for over eight months.

HANNAH

Four years have passed since the events reported about this lady and much has happened since. She suffered greatly from an episode of hepatitis and subsequently from the general feeling of debility and depression. Her husband is fully restored as a caring and devoted spouse, whose next crisis was the sudden and unexpected death of his office manager, a man much younger than himself. Hannah seemed to face this new episode as a confirmation of her own mortality and her husband's need to double his own workload was seen again as a split between them. In response he seemed to show great concern for her and at his request she has been seen by two specialists. Detailed investigation has shown that she is in fact suffering from some organic brain dysfunction and lately her memory has become much worse. She annoys everyone by constant repetition of the same question and has had to stop driving her car. She has twice found herself quite lost and was thoroughly frightened by the experience.

As her doctor, I have accepted that she often makes appointments and forgets to come and see me, turning up unexpectedly at other times. I feel desperately sad for her, as she is very much aware of her own deteriorating condition. None the less last year she had her grandchildren to stay for a couple of weeks and shed many years while they were with her. I still give her occasional prescriptions but mostly just listen to the present situation when she comes to see me. We share desperate feelings of being unable to do very much about the situation and I am all too aware how lonely she feels, despite her caring and concerned husband and family.

'Why don't you listen to me, for a change?'

MARILYN
She was about to leave for Australia at the time of the reported consultation, and there has been no contact since.

NICOLA
Nicola referred herself to the Marriage Guidance Council because one of their Counsellors had been very helpful to her sister. She began regular sessions which resulted in gradual but definite progress. She told me that she found it easier to talk to her (female) counsellor than to anyone else and that she was 'learning to express my anger with my parents'. I saw little of her after this and she seems to have returned to work about 18 months after the reported interview.

VIVIENNE
Vivienne has had a difficult year since her mother's death, but is just surviving. Despite her own problems she involves herself with other people in trouble and manages to help them, often at some cost to herself.

She is still taking sleeping medicine and has severe pre-menstrual symptoms which defy treatment. I see her frequently – two or three times a month – because I feel she needs a good deal of support and it is better for her to have a 'repeat doctor' than too many repeat prescriptions. Her dependence is not burdensome because of her lack of self-pity and her ability to laugh at herself, but the pain is not far below the surface, and she cries a good deal too.

Now that the anniversary of her mother's death has passed, the next hurdle will be Christmas. After this I think she may gradually get back at least to the stage she had reached before her mother's illness, when she was beginning to achieve independence from both drugs and doctor.

Being there

SARAH

It is now just over three years since the reported interviews. There were no contacts with the practice at all for the next three months; an unusually long gap. The next request was for a visit because of an 'increased cough' on New Year's Eve. One of my partners saw her and recorded 'very little wheeziness, chest clear'. There were no clues to the tensions that might have precipitated the call. However, it signalled an abrupt change of doctors. From New Year's Eve she switched to the partner who had visited and continued to see her for the next two years. I felt pretty put out and at a loss to explain why such a change had occurred at that time. What connection did it have to the reported consultations? Any or none? Was my non-availability a significant 'let-down' in the context of the previous interviews? Had she felt similarly 'left out' by her daughter and the new baby? Or was she reverting to her previous long-term pattern of having a woman doctor? She likes to have one doctor, 'her' doctor, and changes her loyalty if the doctor lets her down. Just as abruptly she switched back to seeing me again about six months ago. I had seen her when my partner was away on holiday during August.

She remains needing about one or two consultations each month, mainly coming for 'check-ups' or a further prescription, but often there's a bit extra thrown in as well. She seems to live in a constant fear that others will outdo her and likes to feel she's having 'the best' for herself. We now talk more about these things, and I have learnt a little of her life-long insecurities, originally as a Russian emigrant, and then horrors in Paris during the war when she lost her father, and later her attempts to establish herself on her own in this country. She has never felt settled, either in herself or where she has lived, and constantly tests out those around her. For a persistent hoarseness, when she had become rather depressed, she had lined up her own 'highly recommended' specialist that a friend had recently seen. I understood better this time her need to do things in this way, and she was appreciative. At one time her back became painful after lifting and looking after her 'gorgeous' grandson too much. Generally she tends to be full of praise now for her adopted daughter, and whatever conflicts were surfacing in this area previously, have submerged again.

PEGGY

My expectations that this lady would come back and tell me more were naïve. My partners and I care for her and her family in the usual rather haphazard way. She is rather anxious, and needs attention in a hurry for herself or her children, from whichever doctor is available. However, I think she trusts us. She has only had two slight migraines since the initial interview.

The dependent patient

MISS WATSON

She has been seen very intermittently, but always for the same problems concerning recurrent infection in her 'good' ear and trouble with her hearing-aid. On one occasion she was seen by another doctor in the practice, but ever since then she has insisted on seeing me and was at first very critical of my colleague's clumsiness. She always expresses her gratitude for my skilled care and we get on together in a warm and friendly way. She is brought to the surgery by one of her neighbours and she obviously enjoys the concerned esteem of all the residents in her street. They even arranged a party to celebrate her birthday, to which I was invited.

ANITA

She is still seen frequently and there is only minimal change. However, she does now talk spontaneously about her feelings. For example, she became aware of a tendency to put onto her flatmate some of the feelings she has for her parents. She was able to talk about this with her doctor, though not with the flatmate.

References

Balint, E. and Norell, J.S. (eds) (1973) *Six Minutes for the Patient: Interactions in general practice consultation.* London: Tavistock.

Balint, M. (1957) *The Doctor, His Patient and the Illness.* London: Pitman.

Balint, M. and Balint, E. (1961) *Psychotherapeutic Techniques in Medicine.* London: Tavistock.

Balint, M., Hunt, J., Joyce, D., Marinker, M. and Woodcock, J. (1970) *Treatment or Diagnosis. A study of repeat prescriptions in general practice.* London: Tavistock.

Cartwright, A. (1966) *Patients and their Doctors.* London: Routledge & Kegan Paul.

Cartwright, A. and Anderson, R. (1981) *General Practice Revisited.* London: Tavistock.

Jung, C.G. (1959) *The Archetypes and the Collective Unconscious.* Collected works of C.G. Jung, Vol. 9, p. 284. London: Routledge & Kegan Paul.

Martin, P. and Moulds, A. (1986) Consulting in Comfort. *Pulse* 21 June 1986: 42–6.

Pendleton, D., Schofield, T., Tate, P. and Havelock, P. (1984) *The Consultation: An approach to learning and teaching.* Oxford: Oxford University Press.

Spence, J. (1960) *The Purpose and Practice of Medicine.* London: Oxford University Press.

Tutton, G.R. and Dryden, W. (1983) Dealing with the Emotionally Disturbed Patient. In *Trainee.* Guildford: Update Publications.

Weil, S. (1951) *Waiting on God.* London: Routledge & Kegan Paul.

Woolf, L. (1969) *The Journey Not the Arrival Matters.* London: Hogarth Press.

Index